Informed Consent

Informed Consent

Benjamin J. Brown, M.D.

Printed in the United States of America

The publisher and author will not be responsible for any errors or liable for actions taken as a result of information or opinions expressed in this book. The publisher and author have made every effort to trace the source of data. If they have inadvertently overlooked any, they will be pleased to make the necessary arrangements at the first opportunity.

ISBN 978-0-61543-536-7

Publisher: Informed Advising
Typesetting: www.wordzworth.com
Images and Figures: Benjamin J. Brown
Cover Design: Melanie Bender

Informed Advising
Washington, DC
Informed.Advising@gmail.com
www.informedconsentbook.com

Table of Contents

List of Tables

About the Author

Benjamin Brown spent the first 18 years of his life in the rural Minnesota community of Glenwood where he attended the local public school system from kindergarten through twelfth grade. He completed his first two years of college at the University of Minnesota. While living in Minneapolis he worked as a laboratory assistant at Abbot Northwestern Hospital. After his sophomore year he transferred to Tulane University in order to be closer to his girlfriend at the time, who subsequently became his wife. While living in New Orleans Ben worked as a nurse's assistant at Touro Infirmary and taught MCAT review courses for the Princeton Review. In 2005 he graduated from Tulane University and moved to Dallas where he attended the University of Texas Southwestern Medical School. While in medical school Ben worked with the department of admissions, the office of medical education and served as the student representative on two curriculum committees - experiences which gave him a lot of insight to the U.S. medical education system. During his 4th year of medical school he traveled the country, interviewing at nearly 20 plastic surgery residency programs - an experience that gave him insight into the way residency programs select their residents. In June of 2009 he graduated from medical school, 1st in his class. Following graduation, Ben and his wife moved to Washington, DC. He is currently completing his post-graduate training in Plastic and Reconstructive Surgery.

Acknowledgments

This book is dedicated to my wonderful wife Stephanie who so graciously puts up with me. A special thank you to my family, friends, mentors and colleagues who helped me put together this book.

Stephanie Brown, N.P.
Roderick Brown, M.D.
Renae Brown
Alyssa Gullickson
Kevin Alfortish
Diana Alfortish
Michael Alfortish
Nathan Kirkpatrick
Casey Peterson
Christopher Schwan, M.D.
Darel Jacobsen
Michael Van Hal, M.D.
J. Scott Wright Ed.D.
Benjamin Olson

1 Introduction

Only a fully informed patient with the capacity to understand may give informed consent. For the consent to be considered "informed," a patient must understand the benefits and risks of the procedure, the risks of not having the procedure and the alternative options. If you are considering a career in healthcare, you too should be fully informed of the risks, benefits and alternatives; or more precisely - the sacrifices, rewards and alternative careers.

Healthcare in the United States is a huge industry with many diverse and rewarding careers. In 2007, the United States spent $7,290 per person on healthcare, accounting for 16% of its gross domestic product (GDP) (1). In 2008, there were 14.3 million jobs in the healthcare industry (2). The education and training among these 14.3 million people is highly standardized and regulated. This book is not about the magnificence of medicine; it is an explanation of the system that trains the people who make medicine magnificent.

Careers in the healthcare industry are highly standardized, specialized and inflexible, which means it may cost you extra time and money if you choose to drift through the training system and figure things out as you go. In business, you can do many things with an M.B.A. and change what you do later on in life quite easily. In law, you can do many things with a J.D. and change what you do later on in life quite easily. In healthcare, however, training is standardized and specialized, such that changing your mind or making a poor decision may cost you a lot of time and money.

Some people argue that you cannot plan your life, so you just have to take life as it comes, one day at time. Yes, there are things in life you cannot plan for; however, this does not justify apathy and a reluctance to plan your future. If you are twenty years old, your life expectancy[1] is 81 (3). That means you have about 61 years, 22,265 days or 534,360 hours to live. If you sleep seven hours each night you will spend 155,855 hours sleeping and therefore you will have 378,505 waking hours to enjoy your life. Higher education is expensive and time consuming, and life is short. In order to get the most out of life you need to make the most of your time. In order to make the most of

---

[1]   Which means there is a 50% chance you will die before your 81st birthday and a 50% chance you will die after your 81st birthday.

your time, you need to be efficient. To be efficient, you need to know how to prioritize and plan your time and efforts. In order to prioritize your time and efforts, you need to be informed.

Throughout my medical training, I have heard countless regrets from my colleagues. "I wish I had known X because then I would have done Y;" "I wish I had known X because then I wouldn't have done Z." These regrets were all due to a lack of information. Unfortunately, until the publication of this book, there was no readily available source of the information they needed to make informed decisions. A recent survey administered by the AAMC to first year medical students illustrated how uninformed many of them are. 43% of medical students who started medical school in the fall of 2006 answered "undecided" to the question, *"Are you planning to become board certified in one of the 25 general medical specialties listed below?"(4)*

Due to concern regarding the validity of the question, it was rephrased and presented to 2009's incoming medical students as:

"The following question is about your future career in medicine. In order to practice medicine in the U.S., a physician normally must become board certified in a specialty. Are you planning to become board certified in one of the 25 general specialties listed below?"

This time, only 14% responded "undecided" (4). At graduation, only 7.4% of medical students reported being undecided in 2009, with 89.7% planning on becoming board certified in a medical specialty (5). This suggests that at least one third of matriculating medical students do not understand the basics of the medical education system, much less the nuances of how the system works. First year medical students are at the beginning of 35,000 hours[2] of post-college training, about 10% of their remaining waking life. They are about to spend 10% of their remaining waking hours in the training process, and about to spend an average of $180,000 on tuition and living expenses during medical school, which will cost them $335,000 if paid off over 20 years at a 7% interest rate. When they are finished with residency they will spend approximately 90,000 hours working as a physician, which will account for 25% of their remaining waking life. Yet, astonishingly, many of these students have not begun to understand the sacrifices they are about to make.

In order to make your career choice an informed one, you must have an understanding of the potential rewards and sacrifices. The reward is the career, the sacrifice is the time and money you spend to have that career. To further complicate things, the reward can be bigger or smaller depending on how much you think you will love that career, and the sacrifice can be bigger or smaller depending on how enjoyable or painful the training process will be for you. In order to make the best decision, you need to have an understanding of the rewards and the sacrifices.

---

[2] To put that into perspective; working full-time, year round - or 40 hours per week for 50 weeks - only adds up to 2,000 hours.

Life is short, and even the most direct route to becoming a board certified physician is a long and expensive one. Should you decide to become a physician, you need to be fully informed of the process so you can make good decisions along the way and make the most of your life despite the 35,000-hour time commitment and $180,000 investment. Being efficient and making good decisions along the way can minimize the sacrifices you must make in order to become a physician.

I hope this book will motivate those of you who would have otherwise been too intimidated to consider a career in medicine. I also hope this book will redirect those of you who have been misguided or pressured to pursue a career in medicine, before you invest too much of your time and money. If you decide to pursue a career in medicine, I hope this book will allow you to plan and prioritize your time and efforts so you can get the most out of your life and education.

BENJAMIN J. BROWN

2 Advisors

The difficult thing about advice is that the people who give it to you usually know little about your personality, what you want in life and what motivates you. Furthermore, the outcome of your decision will probably not affect their life in anyway, but it will greatly affect your life. In short, you shouldn't ask advisors to make decisions for you, nor should you let them make decisions for you. What most advisors can offer you is their knowledge and experience, which likely trumps yours. Use them, this book and the resources contained therein to help you become more informed before you make decisions. Also, I encourage you to maintain a healthy level of skepticism, without becoming distrustful. My high school guidance counselor told me I would never get into medical school as a civilian, so I should join the military and try to get into medical school that way. He clearly did not understand the medical education system as there is only one "military medical school," and the application process is no different between civilians and those who are enlisted in the military.

Table 2.1.   *2009 matriculating U.S. Allopathic medical students who answered "very helpful" or "somewhat helpful" regarding advice from the following sources (4)*

Another student or medical student	89.9 %
Premedical advisor	61.5 %
Career/guidance counselor	15.8 %

The advisors common to all of us are likely to be high school guidance counselors, college advisors, pre-med advisors, deans and program directors. I encourage you to listen to all of these people and utilize them to become maximally informed. However, ultimately your decisions are yours to make.

3   College

Higher education is an investment in yourself, it will enrich your life and it may help you to obtain a more rewarding and enjoyable career. Education is, without a doubt, worth going into debt for - so long as you use the time and the money you borrow to become more educated. What many people fail to appreciate is that you pay tuition to be given the opportunity to learn. Whether or not you get your money's worth is your responsibility. You have to study in order to gain the knowledge and skills that will enrich your life and allow you to provide a valuable service to society. Higher education is not about spending money to get a diploma. A diploma is only as valuable as what it represents. What it represents depends on how much you had to learn to earn it. If all you want to do is party, I suggest taking a couple years off before you start college. The last thing you want to do is rack up a lot of debt and bad grades, neither of which will go away easily: bad grades will make it difficult for you to get a good job, the good job that you will need to pay off your debt.

There is nothing wrong with not starting college immediately after high school. Taking time to enjoy your youth and figure out what you want to do with your life is fine, so long as you don't waste this time lounging in your mom's basement. George Bernard Shaw once said, "Life isn't about finding yourself. Life is about creating yourself." Most people find their calling while doing something productive. Whether you start college immediately after high school or not – continue creating yourself.

Think about what you want in life. If you are like most people, you probably don't know what you want in life, even if you think you do at the present time. Nonetheless, the pursuit of happiness and the human condition are beyond the scope of this book. Think about how many years you are willing to spend in school; think about whether or not you enjoy studying.

If you hate school and studying, but want a career in healthcare, I recommend pursuing one of the careers that requires only a 2 year associate's degree such as:

- Registered Nurse (R.N.)
- Paramedic (EMT-P)
- Radiology Tech

- Diagnostic Medical Sonographer
- Surgical Tech or "Scrub"
- Cardiovascular Tech
- Clinical Lab Tech

If you don't mind studying and are very goal oriented, go for the bachelor's degree. With a meaningful[3] bachelor's degree you can move on to do the following:

- Physician (M.D. or D.O.)
- Dentist (D.D.S.)
- Podiatrist (D.P.M.)
- Optometrist (O.D.)
- Veterinarian (D.V.M.)
- Physician Assistant (P.A.)
- Clinical Psychologist (Psy.D.)
- Pharmacist (PharmD)

Fortunately, you don't have to decide which path to take on your first day of college. Although you can minimize the time and money spent in college if you decide which path to take early on. All professional schools have required college courses that must be completed prior to applying for or starting their respective program. It is a good idea to figure out what these required courses are and figure out if there are any pre-requisites for these required courses. This way you can complete them in a timely manner and avoid losing time and spending extra money on college tuition. Required undergraduate courses for most medical, dental, pharmacy and physician assistant schools include: 2 semesters of general chemistry, 2 semesters of physics, 2 semesters of organic chemistry, 4 semesters of biology, 2 semesters of English, and 1 semester of calculus.

Most professional schools also require you to take some type of standardized admission test such as the Graduate Record Examination (GRE), Medical College Admissions Test (MCAT) or Dental Admissions Test (DAT). These admissions tests are extremely important, so you should do your best to take the relevant college courses, utilize review courses and study review books before you take these tests. For example, the MCAT covers general chemistry, physics, organic chemistry and biology. These courses are also required by most medical schools prior to matriculating. Therefore, one should take these courses and then allot time to study for the MCAT before taking the exam.

Ok, so let's say you know you want to get a bachelor's degree, but are not sure what you want to do after college. Yet, you want to keep your options open.

---

[3] By "meaningful" I am referring to a bachelor's degree that represents academic achievement. For example, a bachelor's degree in Geography with a 2.0 GPA probably will not represent academic achievement in the eyes of an employer or admission's committee.

How do you decide which college to go to?

Consider the reputation, success of their graduates, cost, available opportunities, and how well you think you will fit in.

1.   Reputation

Reputation matters. Your academic record will be interpreted by future employers and admissions committees in light of the university where your academic record was earned. A 4.0 GPA from a little known university where the average GPA is 3.8 will be less impressive than a 3.5 GPA from Harvard. By no means do you need to attend an Ivy League institution to be accepted into professional school; what you do need to do is succeed academically wherever you go and make sure your success is evident in your academic record.

2.   Success of their graduates

Find out how successful each institution is at getting their students into professional schools. Many schools boast a higher than 90% professional school acceptance rate among their graduates, but such statistics are often artificially created. An acceptance rate is the percent of students who are accepted out of all those who applied. Universities can maximize this percentage by discouraging all the less than stellar applicants from applying, thereby decreasing the denominator more than the numerator and increasing their "acceptance rate."

Go to: *http://www.aamc.org/data/facts/applicantmatriculant/table2-race.htm* for information on which colleges supply the most students to U.S. allopathic medical schools.

3.   Cost

The total student budget of an institution includes the cost of tuition, fees, room, board, books and supplies. The average total student budgets for the 2009-2010 academic year are listed in Table 3.1. You cannot accurately assess the cost of attending an institution until after you apply, are accepted and given your scholarship and financial aid package. So, before you factor cost into your decision, wait until you receive your scholarship and financial aid package. Private schools often advertise very high tuition costs; however, nearly all students accepted at these institutions receive scholarships. You may think this is strange: if they have so much money to give away in scholarships, why don't they just lower their tuition? One reason is marketing. It is flattering to receive a generous scholarship from an expensive private university. After all, you won't know that everyone else was given that scholarship until after you have moved in, started classes and made friends. Also, be aware of the generous scholarships that are not promised to you each year. What may seem like a reasonable cost for one year may not be so reasonable for the next three.

Remember to consider disparities in living expenses among institutions. For example, your cost of living if you were to attend Carleton College in Northfield, Minnesota will be far less than if you were to attend New York University in Manhattan. Also remember that all the money you borrow will have to be paid back plus interest. If your parents saved up $100,000 for your college education, you don't have to make sure it is all spent by the time you graduate. You may want to have some money tucked away for graduate school, professional school, to start a business, etc. It may be worth spending more to go to a more reputable institution; however, it depends on how much more you will have to spend and how much more reputable the more expensive institution is. It may be worth saving some money and going to a less reputable institution; however, it depends on how much you will save and how much less reputable the more affordable institution is. The variability of cost and reputation among undergraduate institutions is so great that there is no hard and fast rule to help you weigh out those two factors. Ultimately, the individual is more important than the institution. If you find the resources and study hard, you can impress an admissions committee, even if you are at a "less reputable" institution.

Table 3.1.   *Average Undergraduate Total Student Budget for the 2009-2010 academic year (6)*

Public 2-year	$14,285
Public 4-year (In state, on campus)	$19,338
Public 4-year (In state, commuter)	$19,912
Public 4-year (Out of state, on campus)	$30,916
Private 4-year (On campus)	$39,028
Private 4-year (Off campus)	$38,672

4.   Opportunities

You pay tuition to be given the opportunity to learn; the learning part is up to you. It is important that you compare the opportunities available to you among the institutions you are interested in. Let's say you want to major in neuroscience, minor in Russian, play cricket and research synaptic plasticity. You should probably attend an institution that has a neuroscience department, offers Russian and has a cricket league. If you have your sights set on a professional school, you should make sure that the institution offers all of the required courses you will need and has a good track record of getting their graduates accepted.

5.   Fit in

Whether or not you feel like you fit in at an institution is a subjective thing. All you can do is get informed, spend some time there and go with your gut feeling. Life is too short to be miserable. There are so many excellent undergraduate institutions in this country that you should be able to find one that fits both your personality and your career goals.

Combined B.S. / M.D. programs

If you are a high school student and you are confident in your decision to become a physician, you should look into the institutions that offer a combined Bachelor's Degree / Medical Degree (B.S./M.D.) program. At the time this book was published there were 36 institutions offering this program (7). Some of these programs are 6 or 7 year fast-track programs that expedite your way through college and get you to medical school after 2 or 3 years. You are still awarded a bachelor's degree and, in many cases, you do not have to take the MCAT. Some of these programs are 8 years, so they don't necessarily save you time, but you should theoretically be more prepared for medical school and you may get to skip the MCAT.

Accelerated M.D. programs can save you both time and money; fewer years spent in college and medical school means spending less on tuition and less time for your debt to grow. What these programs also offer that may not be immediately apparent is peace of mind. 42,269 people applied to U.S. allopathic medical schools for a position in the entering class of 2009. Only 43.5% (18,390) started allopathic medical school in 2009 (8). These combined programs give you the peace of mind that, as long as you meet all of their expectations, you don't have to worry about that daunting statistic. Before you become too serious about any particular program, be sure to carefully read the details about your "conditional" medical school acceptance.

For a list of these combined programs and their respective websites go to: *http://services.aamc.org/currdir/section3/degree2.cfm?data=yes&program=bsmd.*

What should you major in?

Whatever you want to major in! Professional schools and employers admire students who excel in the sciences, and they admire students who excel in the arts. Bottom line, they admire students who excel, so pick something you will enjoy excelling in. Regardless of what you major in, you will have to take the same pre-requisite courses and entrance exams. If you are not sure what to major in, take a variety of classes, but do your best to take the courses that are pre-requisites for higher-level courses, as this may save you time and money in the future.

COLLEGE

Table 3.2.   *Allopathic (M.D.) Medical School Acceptance Rate by Undergraduate Major (9)*

	Applicants	Matriculants	Matriculation Rate (%)
Humanities	2,041	1,020	50.0
Physical Sciences	4,676	2,329	49.8
Math and Statistics	389	177	45.5
Social Sciences	5,110	2,282	44.7
Biological Sciences	21,630	9,141	42.3
Other	7,185	2,993	41.7
Specialized Health Sciences	1,238	488	39.4
Total	42,269	18,390	43.5

Table 3.3.   *Osteopathic (D.O.) Medical School Acceptance Rate by Undergraduate Major (10, 11)*

	Applicants	Matriculants	Matriculation Rate (%)
Other	1,025	528	52
Life Sciences	10,094	3,947	39
Arts & Humanities	1,138	435	38
Physical Sciences	1,234	457	37
Social Sciences	1,672	580	35
Total	15,163	5947	39

This does not mean that if YOU major in one of the humanities, YOU will be more likely to be accepted by an allopathic medical school. The data in Tables 3.2 and 3.3 does *not* demonstrate a causal relationship between major and medical school acceptance, as there are many confounding variables that are not accounted for. What the data does demonstrate is that people who major in the sciences are not more likely to be accepted to medical school.

Table 3.4.   *Allopathic (M.D.) MCAT Score by Undergraduate Major (9)*

	Avg. Applicant MCAT score	Avg. Matriculant MCAT score
Math and Statistics	30.0 P	32.3 Q
Physical Sciences	29.7 O	32.0 P
Humanities	29.3 Q	31.5 Q
Social Sciences	28.0 P	30.9 Q
Biological Sciences	27.7 O	30.6 P
Other	27.3 O	30.5 P
Specialized Health Sciences	25.5 O	29.5 O
Average	27.9 O	30.8 P

This does not mean that if YOU major in math, YOU will score higher on the MCAT. The data in Table 3.4 does *not* demonstrate a causal relationship between major and MCAT score, as there are many confounding variables that are not accounted for. What the data does demonstrate is that people who major in biology, on average, do not score higher on the MCAT than people who major in one of the humanities.

Will majoring in biology help me perform better in medical school?

Probably not; undergraduate major has not been shown to have a statistically significant correlation with United States Medical Licensing Exam performance (12). Major in something you will enjoy excelling in.

4   The Time Paradigm

par·a·digm [par-uh-dahym, -dim]
—noun

A set of forms all of which contain a particular element, esp. the set of all inflected forms based on a single stem or theme (13).

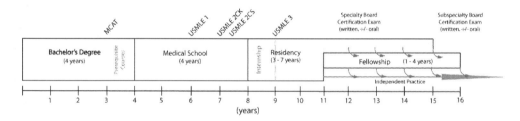

The road to becoming a licensed and board certified physician is a long, complicated and expensive one. It can take anywhere from 11 to 16 years of overtime[4] training after high school.

To become a physician one must first earn a bachelor's degree, which typically takes 4 years. Acceptance to medical school is notoriously competitive, so college students interested in going to medical school usually study more than their peers who are not interested in going to medical school. For most people, medical school is not easy. Most medical students spend about 80 hours per week on medical school activities such as studying, attending lectures and working in the hospital. After medical school, graduates move on to residency. Depending on the specialty, residency can take from 3 to 7 years to complete. The first year of residency is known as internship. To become board certified, one must complete a residency and pass all additional exams for that particular specialty. For example, to become a board certified Internal Medicine physician, one must graduate from medical school, pass all USMLEs, complete a 3-year internal

---

[4] Full-time refers to 40 hours per week. Most medical students, residents and fellows spend nearly 80 hours per week caring for patients and studying.

medicine residency and pass the internal medicine board exam. To become a board certified Thoracic Surgeon, one must graduate from medical school, pass all USMLEs, complete a 5-year general surgery residency, complete a 2-year thoracic surgery fellowship and pass the thoracic surgery board exams. Like medical school, residency is not easy. Most residents approach the legal weekly work-hour limit of 80 hours throughout their residency. Residents do not have to pay tuition, and earn about $50,000 per year, or $12.50 per hour.

The median gross income among men in the United States who work full-time year round is $45,113 (14). The median income among women in the United States who work full-time year round is $35,102 (14). The disparity in income between men and women is beyond the scope of this book to discuss. For the purposes of our discussion below, we will say that the median income of an American who works 40 hours per week for 50 weeks each year is $40,000, or $20 per hour.

The vast majority of working people in the United States are paid based on the number of hours they spend providing a service. The average American who sells 40 hours of their time each week for 50 weeks will receive $40,000. That is $40,000 for 2,000 hours of their time, or $20.00 per hour. Of that $40,000 paid to them by their employer, they will likely have to pay about $5,000 in income taxes, leaving them with $35,000. There are 8,760 hours in a year. If one sleeps 7 hours each night, they are left with 6,205 hours per year during which they are awake. If one sells 2,000 hours to their employer, they are left with 4,205 waking hours per year that are still owned by them. Therefore, the average American owns 4,205 waking hours and $35,000 of net pay each year.

Let's call the average American "Pat." If a bank loans Pat $40,000 he/she would be indebted one year of work to that bank, one year's income - right? Wrong, Pat would be indebted more than 1 year of full-time work because he/she would have to pay back that loan plus its interest with his/her post-tax income of $35,000. So, in reality, a $35,000 loan - or even less, considering the cost of interest - is equivalent to Pat working full-time for one year. On the other hand, if Pat won $40,000 playing the lottery, Pat would be left with about $35,000 after taxes and he/she could take the year off.

The paradigm is that $40,000 of gross income, $35,000 of net income and 2,000 hours of work are roughly equivalent for the average American.

$40,000 gross income = $35,000 net income = 2,000 hours

To become a Registered Nurse via the Associate's degree pathway will take you about 3,200 hours. The average total student budget per year for these students is $14,285 (6). Therefore, after 2 years, their debt is $28,570. Should you decide to work while attending nursing school, you could lessen your debt, assuming you don't allow this extra work to extend the amount of time you spend in nursing school. To keep things consistent and simple, let's assume you don't work – you spend 1,600 hours per year studying and training to become a nurse, and the other 4,605 waking hours of the year are yours to spend doing something other than studying, training or working for money.

To become an R.N. via the Associate's degree pathway you will spend about 3,200 hours studying and training.[5] You will likely need to borrow or spend about $28,570 to cover tuition and living expenses during these two years. This is nearly equivalent to 2.5 years: the 1.6 years of time you spent studying and training plus the 0.9-year equivalent you owe your student loan lender.

Table 4.1.   *Registered Nurse (R.N.) via the Associate's degree pathway*

	Hours	Debt/Cost	Year Equivalents	Hour Equivalents
Nursing School	-3,200	-$28,570	-2.42	-4,840

To become a high school teacher you will have to earn a bachelor's degree. If you attend college full-time, this endeavor will take you 4 years, or 6,400 hours studying and training.[6] The average total student budget for 4-year colleges and universities is about $25,000 per year, or $100,000 over four years. Therefore, to become a high school teacher you will have to invest the equivalent of 6 years of full-time work.

Table 4.2.   *High School Teacher*

	Hours	Debt/Cost	Year Equivalents	Hour Equivalents
College	-6,400	-$100,000	-6.06	-12,120

To become a dentist you will first have to earn a bachelor's degree. If you attend college full-time, this will take you 4 years. In order to be competitive for acceptance into dental school, you will likely spend more than 40 hours per week studying, doing research and volunteering. However, to keep it simple and consistent, we will neglect that extra time. After college you will need to attend dental school. In dental school you are likely to spend about 60 hours per week for 48 weeks each year studying and training to become a dentist. The average annual cost of tuition and fees for in-state students and out-of-state students is about $27,000 and $42,000, respectively (15). For our calculations we will use $35,000 per year for tuition plus $15,000 per year for living expenses. After dental school, further residency training is optional, so you have the option to start practicing independently without completing a dental residency.

---

[5]   2 years x 40 wks/yr x 40 hrs/wk = 3,200 hours
[6]   4 years x 40 wks/yr x 40 hrs/wk = 6,400 hours

Table 4.3. *Dentist (D.D.S. or D.M.D.)*

	Hours	Debt/Cost	Year Equivalents	Hour Equivalents
College	-6,400	-$100,000	-6.06	-12,120
Dental School	-11,520	-$200,000	-11.47	-22,940
Total	-17,920	-$300,000	-17.53	-35,060

To become a physician you first have to earn a bachelor's degree. If you attend college full-time, this will take you 4 years. In order to be competitive for acceptance into medical school you are likely to spend far more than 40 hours per week studying, doing research and volunteering. However, to keep it simple and consistent we will neglect that extra time. After college you will need to attend medical school. In medical school, you are likely to spend about 80 hours per week, for 48 weeks each year, studying and training to become a physician. The average total student budget for medical students is about $45,000 per year, or $180,000 over four years (16). After medical school you will need to attend residency in order to become board certified and gain the experience you need to be a competent physician. Depending on the specialty, residency and fellowship can take anywhere from three to eight years. We will use five years in our example. Most residencies will consume about 80 hours per week of your time for 50 weeks each year. The silver lining is that you will be paid about $50,000 per year during residency, $12.50 per hour, and you no longer have to pay tuition. Therefore, your net income during residency will be about $40,000 per year, or $10 per hour. So, unlike medical school, where you are taking out loans to work 2 full-time jobs, in residency you work 2 full-time jobs and get paid for one.

Table 4.4. *Physician (M.D. or D.O.)*

	Hours	Debt/Cost	Year Equivalents	Hour Equivalents
College	-6,400	-$100,000	-6.06	-12,120
Medical School	-15,360	-$180,000	-12.82	-25,640
Residency	-20,000	+$200,000	-4.29	-8,580
Total	-41,760	-$80,000	-23.17	-46,340

By the time you finish residency and finally start practicing medicine independently after 13 years of post-secondary training you will have worked and indebted yourself the equivalent of 23 years of full-time work. Moreover, you will likely continue to work 1.5 times as much most Americans for the rest of your career. In 2007, physicians from over 20 specialties were asked how many hours per week they generally work – the average was 59.6 hours per week (17).

Why does it have to take so long?

There are no shortcuts to gaining the knowledge and experience you need to be a competent physician; you need to put in the time to get the experience. There are, however, certain inefficiencies in the medical education system. It could be argued that you don't need four years of undergraduate education before starting medical school. Medical school and residency training also have inefficiencies that vary among schools, specialties and programs. To some degree, residents in a program can only progress as fast as the weakest resident in the program. Let's say you are a third year general surgery resident and there is a patient who needs their gallbladder removed. The attending physician and a resident will probably remove the gallbladder via a procedure known as a laparoscopic cholecystectomy. If the fifth-year is a weak resident and doesn't feel comfortable with this operation, they will do more of the operation and the third-year resident will do less. Therefore, the third-year resident's opportunity to learn an operation is postponed due to the weak senior resident who should feel comfortable with a laparoscopic cholecystecomy at that point in their training. If the fifth-year resident feels comfortable with this operation, they will let the third-year resident do more and therefore learn more. Medical training can be viewed as a cumulative advantage or disadvantage. The more you learn to do at an early stage, the better you become earlier in your training, and you are then given more opportunities to learn and are able to take advantage of more opportunities to learn - and you progress faster. If an attending physician trusts you to do more complicated things early in your training, they may give you the opportunity to do more complicated things sooner. You will thus be able to master more complicated things earlier, and they will then trust you to do even more, and so on, such that your competence and responsibilities increase exponentially. On the other hand, medical training can also be a cumulative disadvantage. If you lack confidence in yourself or your attending physicians don't trust you, you may be denied many opportunities, causing you to learn less and ultimately progress much more slowly.

Because there is no shortcut to gaining the experience you need to be a competent physician, decreasing resident work hours from 80 hours per week to 60 hours per week is a terrible idea. If such a change occurs, residency training would have to become years longer in order to get the same experience. Making physician training longer will further increase student debt loads and decrease the number of years physicians are able to work after they are trained. It will also increase the number of physicians in training and decrease the physician workforce.

It is important to realize that life doesn't stop while you are a medical student or a resident. The mundane aspects of life continue; you still have to go grocery shopping, do laundry, pay bills, clean your house, exercise, get your oil changed, etc. You just have to fit these mundane tasks into your limited amount of free time. Unfortunate events also still happen; your significant other can still break up with you, your car can break down, a family member can become ill, you can become ill, your identity can be stolen, etc. You just have to deal with these unfortunate events in your limited amount of free time amidst your inflexible schedule.

Many things in life are easily postponed until after you are done with residency. Ski resorts, golf courses and most vacation destinations will still be there when you are done with residency. Unfortunately, the ability to have children of your own may not be there when you are done with residency. Infertility is an evil reality that sneaks up on many couples who postpone having children until after residency – when they expect to have more time and money.

Infertility is defined as the inability of a couple to conceive after one year of regular intercourse without contraception. Primary infertility refers to a woman or man who has never been pregnant or contributed to a pregnancy, respectively. Secondary infertility refers to a woman or man who has a history of one or more previous pregnancies. Fecundability is the probability that a couple will conceive within one menstrual cycle; this is about 25% for a normal couple (18). Sterility is defined as the complete inability to conceive a child naturally. About 1% of couples are sterile (19). Unlike infertility, sterility does not appear to increase with age (19).

With increasing maternal age comes decreasing fertility rates, increased rates of miscarriage and stillbirth, increased rates of chromosomal abnormalities and increased hypertensive complications during pregnancy (20). Table 4.5 illustrates the decreasing ability of women to give birth to a normal, healthy child as they age. The fertility statistics in Table 4.5 are derived from couples with no known fertility problems.

Table 4.5.   *Risks of Delayed Childbearing (18, 19, 21-25)*

Maternal Age	Ability to conceive by:			Miscarriage Rate	% Down's Syndrome at live birth	% with any chromosomal abnormality at live birth	Your age when child is 18 years old [7]
	12 months	18 months	24 months				
18					0.067		37
19					0.067		38
20					0.068	0.2	39
21					0.068		40
22	92%	95.4%	97%		0.069		41
23				10%	0.071		42
24					0.072		43
25					0.075	0.2	44
26					0.078		45
27					0.082		46
28					0.088		47
29					0.096		48
30	86%	91.2%	93.7%		0.107	0.3	49
31					0.122		50
32				12%	0.144		51
33					0.175		52
34					0.220		53
35					0.284	0.5	54
36					0.376		55
37	82%	87.9%	91.2%	18%	0.503		56
38					0.677		57
39					0.900		58
40					1.176	1.5	59
41					1.493	1.9	60
42	71%			34%	1.852	2.3	61
43					2.222	3.0	62
44					2.564	3.8	63
45	13%			53%	2.857	5.0	64

Increasing paternal age carries a very small, but nevertheless slightly, increased risk of autosomal dominant diseases such as Marfan's syndrome and achondroplasia (20). Male

---

[7]   If you or your partner conceives a child at 18 years old, they will give birth about 9 months later and the child will turn 18 years old 18 years after their birth – about 19 years after conception.

fertility is less age dependent; however, it does appear to decline somewhat in the late 30s. The infertility rate of couples composed of two 35 year olds is 18% (19). The infertility rate of couples composed of a 35 year old woman and a 40 year old man is 28%, suggesting that male infertility increases with age as well (19).

Unfortunately, assisted reproductive technologies are not a perfect solution for the older couple who are unable to conceive. Ovulation induction and intrauterine insemination have a pregnancy rate of 5% or less per cycle in women older than 40 years of age, with unexplained infertility (26). Moreover, there is accumulating evidence that children conceived by assisted reproductive technologies are at increased risk of cognitive deficiencies (27).

Depending on how many children you want to have and how old you will be when you finish residency, it may not be a problem to postpone having children until you are finished with your training. If you want to have four children, but will be 35 years old by the time you finish your training, you will probably have to start having children while you are in medical school and residency.

When does one have children during medical school, residency or fellowship?

There is no perfect time to have children during this process, but there are "better" times. Usually, the fourth year of medical school is the least intense year. So, having a child at the beginning of your fourth year is a good idea, if you and your partner are fortunate enough to be able to time such events. Remember that your child will not disappear or pause in their development while you are in residency. The hardest year of residency is typically the first year of residency, your internship, which inconveniently follows your fourth year of medical school. The duration and intensity of your residency training will depend on the specialty you go into and the program where you train. Many students who want to have children during medical school and residency take a year or two off to do research. This is a good option, as one's schedule is much more flexible while doing research than while they are caring for patients. The downside to taking time off to do research is that it prolongs the process. Moreover, when you return to the clinical side of medicine to finish your residency, your children will still be there and will still need you.

How does one have children while in medical school, residency or fellowship?

Support. It is nearly impossible for a single mother or father to care for a child while they are working 80 hours per week and earning $10 per hour. To make it work, you will require some combination of support and more time. Support can come from your significant other, if they have the time. Support can also come from your family or friends, if they live close by, or a nanny, if you can afford it. More time and a more flexible schedule can be achieved by going into a less demanding specialty. Such specialties include: dermatology, radiology, pathology, ophthalmology, emergency medicine, anesthesiology, physical medicine & rehabilitation and psychiatry. Some of these, such as dermatology and radiology, are very competitive, with match rates of 60% and 74%, respectively (28). This means you cannot "plan" on becoming a dermatologist, as 40% of those who apply and interview for dermatology residency positions do not end up in dermatology. For information on medical specialties, see chapter 13, and for more information on residency match rates by specialty, see chapter 16.

If you want to be a pediatric surgeon and you want to have 3 children by the time you are 35 years old, you will need to plan accordingly. You can have children during medical school, residency and fellowship. Regardless of how accommodating your medical school, residency or fellowship program is, however, you will still need to invest a lot of time in yourself throughout your training, as there is no shortcut to gaining the knowledge and experience you need to be a competent pediatric surgeon. In order to have sufficient time to invest in your career you will need to have help raising your children. This support can come from your partner, your family, daycare or a nanny. Therefore, you need to consider these factors when you choose a medical school and when you make your residency rank list.

This is difficult. While you are a medical student and a resident you will have to work a lot and you will have little control over your hours, which means you will have to rely on others to help raise your children. Moreover, unless you are independently wealthy or have a generous family, you won't have much money. If your partner can make up for the time you don't have without jeopardizing the income your family needs to survive, great. If you are relying on your partner's income to survive and your partner has to work a lot as well, then you will need to find a nanny or send your children to daycare – which costs money.

The cost of living where you receive your residency training can make a huge difference in your ability to start a family early. Regardless of where you train, your resident salary will be about $50,000, but $50,000 will go a lot further in Winston-Salem, North Carolina than in San Francisco, California.

In addition to considering the location and cost of living, you also need to make sure the residency program is well respected and has a good track record of getting its graduates into quality fellowships.

As you can see, one must plan accordingly and hope for the best in the residency and subspecialty matches.

Fortunately, once you are a licensed and board certified physician you are likely to have excellent job security and transferability. Let's say you have a twin sister. After college, you go to medical school and she goes on to graduate school to earn a Master of Business Administration (MBA). Eleven years after college graduation you are a board certified general surgeon with two years of experience and she is an MBA who has spent the last ten years working her way up the corporate ladder at business X. After ten years of working her way up the corporate ladder, business X comes on hard times and is dissolved. Your sister has an MBA and ten years of experience at business X, so hopefully business Y will offer her a good job; however, her ten years of service at business X are not necessarily transferrable to business Y.

You, however, are in a different position.

Let's say after two years of practicing general surgery at hospital X, your mother becomes ill and you decide to move closer to your family. Fortunately, your experience and training is easily transferable, since you are a licensed and board certified general surgeon. All those exams you had to take along the way now provide you with an objective, well-defined and widely accepted indication of your competence to provide a complex service to society.

The greatest insecurity that comes with being a physician is the highly regulated market in which physicians work. The healthcare industry is not a free-market. Physician reimbursements are determined by the government and by insurance companies, not the market. You may have 43,360 hours of post-high-school training and owe $300,000 in student loans, but the government and insurance companies will ultimately decide to pay you whatever they feel is appropriate. For more information on the finances of becoming a physician see chapter 5.

5   MD = Massive Debt

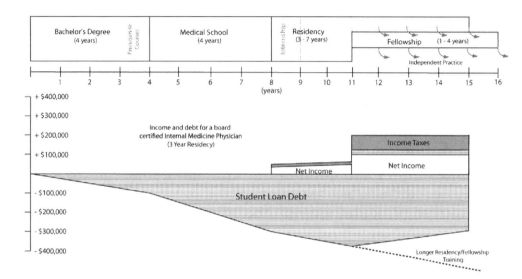

Like it or not, money is an inescapable reality. Unless you are independently wealthy or have a generous family, you will likely have to have to borrow a significant amount of money in order to become a physician. Hopefully, after you finish residency, you won't have to struggle to pay off your student loan debt. Nonetheless, medicine is not as financially rewarding as it once was, so you should avoid using older physicians as a marker of how much money you will make. For over a decade, physician reimbursements, on average, have been decreasing while college and medical school tuition has continued to increase. Furthermore, student loan interest rates have continued to rise and most people can no longer defer student loan payments during residency.[8]

Say you are $100,000 in debt after college. Because you will probably go to college regardless of whether or not you go medical school, the burden of accruing college debt is a moot point. However, what does matter is that it will be another decade or so

---

[8]   The ability to defer your loans during residency depends on your economic circumstances and the composition of your loans. Most residents nowadays are not able to defer their loans throughout residency.

before you can start paying that debt off, should you decide to become a physician. Let's assume that the government will allow you to defer your college debt during medical school. While in deferment, the government pays the interest on your loans, which prevents the principal from increasing during that time period. Deferment is not to be confused with forbearance. When your loans are in forbearance, you do not have to make any payments; however, the accrued interest is added to your principal each year. Assuming you are able to defer your college debt throughout medical school, it will still be $100,000 after medical school. Unfortunately, during residency, when you can no longer defer that debt – your loans from college and medical school will accrue interest and grow accordingly.

For the 2009-2010 academic year, the median cost of tuition and fees for public and private medical schools was $24,384 and $43,002 per year, respectively (16).[9] This does not include the cost of rent, utilities, food, transportation, health insurance, books, professional attire, licensing exams or residency interview expenses. So, let's say your medical school tuition is $30,000 per year and you borrow an extra $15,000 per year for living expenses – totaling $45,000 per year. Each semester in medical school you will receive a financial aid package made up of a few different loans. Some of these will hopefully be subsidized, which means the government pays the interest while you are in medical school - like deferment. Let's assume that one third of your loans are subsidized. The other two thirds are accruing interest while you are in medical school. If you borrow $22,500 bi-annually and two-thirds of this accrues interest compounded bi-annually at 3.5%, you will have $200,527 of debt from medical school at graduation. Your total student loan debt for both college and medical school will then be $300,527.

Are most medical school graduates $300,527 in debt? No, but that is not the point. The point is, if you attend an averaged priced college and an average priced medical school, it will cost about $280,000 to educate you. Whether you pay for it with student loans, your parents pay for it, or the military pays for it – it still costs a lot, and it costs a lot more if you have to pay it back with interest.

Fortunately, you won't have to pay tuition during residency. In fact, you will get paid during residency. The mean stipend, or salary, of interns (R1s, PGY-1s) for the 2009-2010 academic year was $47,458 before taxes and benefits were withheld (29). This stipend increases by roughly $2000 each year such that the average stipend for a PGY-6, resident or fellow, was $57,871 (29). Depending on your financial responsibilities during residency, you may be able to start making payments on your student loans. In the past, residents were able to defer payment of their loans until after residency. This was great, because their student loans didn't get larger while they were in residency. Unfortunately, this option is no longer available to most people. Residents are

---

[9] For a list of allopathic medical schools and their respective tuition costs go to https://services.aamc.org/tsfreports/

able to forbear repayment of their student loans while in residency and fellowship. Forbearance is nice in that residents don't have to stress out about making payments each month. However, the loans quietly grow at an exponential rate throughout residency.

In the past, before 80-hour workweek regulations were instituted, most residents were able to moonlight in emergency departments to make extra money during residency. Nowadays, fewer residents are able to moonlight due to 80-hour workweek regulations and other rules instituted by their residency program.

If you paid for college and medical school yourself with student loans, it will continue to grow until you can pay it off.

Starting with a debt of $300,527 at an annual percentage interest rate of 7% compounded biannually at 3.5%.

If you make no payments during a 3-year residency you will be $369,425 in debt at the end of your residency.

If you make no payments during a 6-year residency you will be $454,118 in debt at the end of your residency.

If you make payments of $1,753 per month, or $21,037 per year, to pay off the accruing interest during residency, your debt will be still be $300,527 at the end of residency. However, you will have spent $63,111 over the course of a 3 year residency or $126,222 over the course of a 6-year residency to keep your debt from growing. Though paying off the interest during residency is the responsible thing to do, coming up with $21,037 each year from your net pay of $40,000 may be quite difficult.

It's daunting isn't it: to think that you will be about 30 years old and in massive debt, even though you spent the past decade working harder than most of your peers?

So, you are done with residency. You are a board certified physician in a specialty you enjoy, and it is finally time to make the big bucks - right?

Income varies greatly by specialty (see table 13.1 for details). For purposes of discussion, let's say you are a pediatrician who is married with 2 children and lives in California. The median gross income of a pediatrician is $202,832 (30). After income tax, you will be left with $139,372 per year, $11,614 per month. These figures are calculated assuming a federal Income tax structure as described in table 5.2, with the California state income tax rate of 6.6%, Social Security tax rate of 6.2% and Medicare tax rate of 1.45%. You can go to *www.paycheckcity.com* to get an idea of what your net pay would be for different incomes, states of residence, marital status, number of children, etc.

You may be shocked by how much is lost in taxes. For decades, the United States federal income tax rate has been progressive. This means that the higher your adjusted gross income is the higher percentage of your income you will pay in federal income tax.

Table 5.1. *In 2010 for a single person with an annual adjusted gross income of (31)*

Greater than	Less Than	Federal Income Tax Paid
	$6,050	none
$6,050	$10,425	10%
$10,425	$36,050	$437.50 plus 15% of the remaining balance
$36,050	$67,700	$4,281.25 plus 25% of the remaining balance
$67,700	$84,450	$12,193.75 plus 27% of the remaining balance
$84,450	$87,700	$16,716.25 plus 30% of the remaining balance
$87,700	$173,900	$17,691.25 plus 28% of the remaining balance
$173,900	$375,700	$41,827.25 plus 33% of the remaining balance
$375,700		$108,421.25 plus 35% of the remaining balance

Table 5.2. *In 2010 for a married person filing jointly with an annual adjusted gross income of (31)*

Greater than	Less Than	Federal Income Tax Paid
	$13,750	none
$13,750	$24,500	10%
$24,500	$75,750	$1,075 plus 15% of the remaining balance
$75,750	$94,050	$8,762.50 plus 25% of the remaining balance
$94,050	$124,050	$13,337.50 plus 27% of the remaining balance
$124,050	$145,050	$21,437.50 plus 25% of the remaining balance
$145,050	$217,000	$26,687.50 plus 28% of the remaining balance
$217,000	$381,400	$46,833.50 plus 33% of the remaining balance
$381,400		$101,085.50 plus 35% of the remaining balance

Pediatrics is a three-year residency, allowing your $300,527 of debt to grow to $369,425 by the time you are done. If you plan on paying off $369,425 of student loan debt at an APR of 7% over 20 years, you will have to spend $34,368 per year, or $2,864 per month, of your *net* income for 20 years. If you are a pediatrician who is married with 2 children, living in California with a gross income of $202,832, you will be left with $105,004 per year, or $8,750 per month, of post-tax and post-loan payment income to get a late start on buying a home, putting money away for your children's education and investing for your retirement. After residency forbearance and

20 years of payments, what started off as $280,000 in student loans will end up costing you $687,360 due to that 7% interest rate.

To continue our discussion, let's say you are a cardiologist who is married with 2 children and living in California. The median gross income of a cardiologist is $398,034 (30). After income taxes you will be left with $248,219 per year, or $20,685 per month. Cardiology training consists of a three-year internal medicine residency followed by a three-year cardiology fellowship, allowing your $300,527 of debt to grow to $454,118 by the time you are done. If you plan on paying off $454,118 of student loan debt at an APR of 7% over 20 years you will have to spend $42,252 per year, or $3,521 per month, of your *net* income for 20 years. You will thus be left with $205,967 per year, or $17,164 per month, of post-tax and post-loan payment income to make a late start on buying a home, putting money away for your children's education and investing for your retirement. After residency forbearance and 20 years of payments, what started off as $280,000 in student loans will end up costing you $845,040 due to that 7% interest rate.

You will probably *not* be able to deduct the interest on your student loans from your income taxes. The U.S. tax code allows you to deduct a maximum of $2,500 per year if your modified adjusted gross income is less than $115,000. If your modified adjusted gross income is greater than $145,000, you cannot deduct any of your student loan interest (32).

If you were to start a business, you could deduct nearly all of your expenses, including: computers, rent and educational conferences. For unclear reasons, you cannot deduct the cost of becoming a physician: not your tuition or even the interest on the money you borrowed to pay your tuition.

Student loans are exempt from bankruptcy, so, in case you were wondering, you can't graduate from medical school, file bankruptcy and start even.

The cost of tuition, the length of training and the U.S. tax code places physicians in a deceptive financial situation. One pays more in taxes if one makes a large sum of money over a short period of time than if one were to make a moderate amount of money over a longer period of time. Physicians spend over a decade of time which could be spent earning, saving and investing. Instead they are taking on more debt, debt which isn't tax deductible. Then, when they are finished and finally have an income, they are taxed heavily and must repay their debt with what remains of their income. Because the training process takes so long, physicians have less time in which to invest for their retirement.

You might be wondering why physicians don't just charge more for their services. The truth is, medicine is not a free market. Physicians are not simply paid the amount they ask for their services. The insurance companies and the government decide how much physicians are reimbursed for each service. This makes it very difficult for physicians to adjust in an ever-changing market. In most other industries, if operating costs increase, the business can shift some of that cost to the consumer. If a physician's malpractice insurance premiums increase or the property taxes on their building increase, physicians cannot simply adjust the fee they charge patients, because the insurance companies and the government have to agree.

When the government and insurance companies talk about reducing physician reimbursements by "20%," that doesn't mean that a physician's gross income will go from $200,000 to $160,000 – it will most likely decrease by much, much more. Let's say Dr. Smith, an internal medicine physician, spends 15 minutes caring for a Medicare patient in clinic and bills Medicare $100 for this service. From that visit, Dr. Smith's profit margin is about 40%: $60 to cover his overhead and $40 profit. Medicare typically pays about 60 cents on the dollar, if you are lucky, which is why most physicians barely break even caring for Medicare patients. The 20% decrease in physician reimbursements will likely be 20% of that $60, so Dr. Smith will now be reimbursed only $48 dollars for that visit, which is less than it cost Dr. Smith to see the patient. Therefore, Dr. Smith will *spend* $12 to see that Medicare patient. This is generous of Dr. Smith, but it is unsustainable. This "20%" decrease in reimbursements won't simply bring Dr. Smith's gross income of $200,000 down to $160,000; it will put Dr. Smith out of business.

Aside from interest groups and lobbyists, the only defense physicians have against unfair reimbursements from Medicare, Medicaid and insurance companies is to refuse to provide services to the constituents of these organizations until they agree to fair reimbursements. Such a refusal is, in fact, legal - though it may seem morally and ethically wrong. Then again, isn't it morally and ethically wrong to expect a group of honest, hard-working citizens to operate their business at a loss?

There has been discussion that the government might coerce physicians to provide care to Medicare and Medicaid patients by withholding their medical license unless they agree to care for a certain number of these patients. If the government continues to reimburse physicians poorly or further decreases reimbursements for caring for these patients, physicians will be placed in an extremely difficult financial situation. They will be loaded with debt, taxed heavily and trained to provide a service which they may not be able to make much, if any, money providing.

What about outcome based reimbursements?

As of 2009, most physicians are paid based on the services they provide to patients, which is known as "fee-for-service." Some people argue that this creates an incentive for physicians to provide more services to patients regardless of whether or not it will improve that patient's outcome. Outcome based physician reimbursements is based on the idea that physicians will be paid on the basis of patients' outcomes rather than the services they provide. This is a great idea in theory, but a terrible idea from a practical standpoint. Most "outcomes" in medicine cannot be measured, quantified or standardized. How do you measure and standardize a 64 year old gentleman with metastatic lung cancer, type 2 diabetes mellitus and depression for whom you optimize his quality of life for 3 months before he dies? What is the "outcome" for this patient? What does "optimized" mean for *this* patient? What would have happened to him if he had never seen a physician? What was the effect of the physician's interventions? Were they the correct interventions? Who decides what is "correct"?

You see a patient in clinic who has insulin dependent type 2 diabetes mellitus and hypertension. In order to be reimbursed, you need to lower their blood pressure and their hemoglobin A1C level. To lower their blood pressure you could use many medications. Let's say you use a diuretic as a first line anti-hypertensive medication in this diabetic patient. Their blood pressure is better, should you be reimbursed? Some studies would suggest that you should have used an ACE inhibitor in this patient with diabetes, not a diuretic. Let's say there is a system in place that catches your "error" and therefore doesn't reimburse you. But what if you know that ACE inhibitors are typically the first line anti-hypertensive agent for most diabetics, but you also know that in the past ACE inhibitors have caused hyperkalemia in *this* patient which led to symptomatic cardiac dysrhythmias. You weighed the risks and benefits and decided a diuretic was best for this patient.

Physicians spend their day gathering data and making decisions as fast as they can, usually without compromising patient safety. One supervising physician cannot gather the same data and analyze the decisions and outcomes of hundreds of physicians. In fact, it would probably take one physician to review the data, decisions and outcomes of each physician. To gather the same data, analyze it, make a decision and follow-up on the outcome will take the reviewing physician nearly the same amount of time as the practicing physician. Therefore, in order to institute outcome-based reimbursements, the United States would need twice as many physicians, one group to take care of patients and the other to supervise them. Moreover, the supervising physicians would have to be omniscient in order to judge the work of the mortal physicians.

Medicine is an art; each patient must be treated individually. Patient care cannot be standardized and outcomes can rarely be measured and quantified for an individual patient.

What about non-compliant patients?

Lowering blood pressure, lowering cholesterol levels, and maintaining good glucose control all depend more on patient compliance than physician effectiveness. Yes, a good physician will develop a treatment plan that a given patient is most likely to be compliant with, but ultimately the outcome rests on the patient's compliance. Outcome based reimbursements would create a disincentive to care for non-compliant patients.

What is the net hourly wage of physicians in 2009 after being adjusted for hours spent training and student loan debt?

$$\text{Adjusted Net Hourly Wage} = \frac{(\text{Net Annual Income x Years Worked}) + (\text{Residency Income}) - (\text{Student Debt})}{(\text{Avg hours worked per week x weeks worked per year x years worked}) + (\text{Hours Training})}$$

In order to make this calculation we will neglect inflation of the U.S. dollar by assuming that inflation of the U.S. dollar will increase at the same rate as the purchasing power of the U.S. dollar decreases. We will also assume that physician incomes keep pace with inflation, and that tuition costs, student loan interest rates, resident stipends, physician reimbursements and the U.S. income tax structure are as described above and do not change.

The median gross income among internal medicine physicians is $205,441 (30). The median net income for an internist who is married with two children living in California is then $140,939. Internal medicine is a three-year residency, so throughout their residency they will earn about $120,000[10] and spend about 33,760 hours training after high school. The total cost of training including interest, forborn for three years and paid off over 20 years, as explained above, is $687,260. One study reported that the average hours worked per week by practicing Internal medicine physicians was 57 hours per week (33). Another study reported the mean to be 55.5 hours per week (34). We will use 56 hours per week and assume they work 48 weeks per year. If they finish residency at 29 years old and retire at 65, they will work for 36 years at that median income.

[(140,939 x 36) + (120,000) – (687,260)] / [(56 x 48 x 36) + (33,760)] = $34.53
The adjusted net hourly wage for an internal medicine physician is then $34.53

The median gross income among general surgeons is $340,000 (30). The median net income of a general surgeon who is married with two children living in California is then $216,315. General surgery is a five-year residency, so throughout residency they will earn about $200,000 and spend about 41,760 hours training after high school. The total cost of training including interest, forborn for five years and paid off over 20 years, will end up costing $788,880. Practicing general surgeons work an average of 60 hours per week (33). We will assume they work 48 weeks per year. If they finish residency at 31 years old and work until they are 65 years old they will work for 34 years at that median income

---

[10]   A net income of $40,000 per year times 3 years = $120,000

$$[(216,315 \times 34) + (200,000) - (788,880)] / [(60 \times 48 \times 34) + (41,760)] = \$48.44$$
The adjusted net hourly wage for a general surgeon is then $48.44

Variables that will decrease this adjusted net hourly wage include: a shorter career, increased taxation, decreased income, working more hours for the same or less pay, spending more than average on tuition, spending more time training and decreased resident pay.

Variables that will increase this adjusted net hourly wage include: a longer career, decreased taxation, increased income, working fewer hours for the same or more pay, spending less than average on tuition, having less debt, paying off your debt early and increased resident pay.

Let's say that you are a senior in high school and you can't decide whether you should be a physician, dentist, high school teacher or a registered nurse. From a purely financial standpoint, let's see if it is worth becoming a physician.

The median gross income among general dentists who work full-time in a group practice is $220,000 (35). The median net income for a general dentist who is married with two children living in California is then $149,681. General dentists who work full-time in a group practice with partners work an average of 38 hours per week, 1,727 hours per year (35). Dentists spend about 17,920 hours training after high school. The total cost of training, if you attend averaged priced institutions and pay off your debt over 20 years at a 7% interest rate, is $558,216. If you finish dental school at 26 years old and retire at 65 years old you will work for 39 years.

$$[(149,681 \times 39) - (558,216)] / [(1,727 \times 39) + (17,920)] = \$61.91$$
The adjusted net hourly wage for a general dentist is then $61.91

The median gross income among high school teachers, including the value of benefits but excluding their pension, is about $50,000 (36). The median net income for a high school teacher who is married with two children living in California is then $42,791. Teachers spend about 6,400 hours training after high school. The total cost of training if you attend an averaged priced institution and pay off your debt over 20 years at a 7% interest rate is $186,072. At this income, you will be able to deduct the interest on your student loans from your income taxes (these savings are not accounted for in the calculation below). High school teachers have about 10 weeks off each summer, 2 weeks off during Christmas, 1 week off for spring break and 1 week of personal paid time off. Therefore, high school teachers who work full-time work an average of 40 hours per week for 38 weeks each year. Yes, teachers spend time "off the clock" preparing for class, correcting papers, etc. However, physicians, dentists and nurses also spend time "off the clock" reading, studying, going to conferences, etc. If you finish college at

22 years old and retire at 65 years old, you will work for 43 years. Most teachers also receive a pension. We will assume your gross annual pension, including the value of benefits, is $40,000, which is a net pension of $35,507. If you die at 80 years old, you will receive this pension for 15 years.

$$[(42{,}791 \times 43) + (35{,}507 \times 15) - (186{,}072)] \,/\, [(40 \times 38 \times 43) + (6{,}400)] = \$30.47$$

The adjusted net hourly wage for a high school teacher is then $30.47

Though the gross income of an internal medicine physician is 4 times that of a high school teacher, the adjusted net hourly wage of an internal medicine physician is only 1.13 times that of a high school teacher.

The median gross income of a registered nurse is $62,450 (37). The median net income of a registered nurse who is married with two children and lives in California is then $51,787. To become a registered nurse via the associate's degree route takes 2 years, about 3,200 hours of training. The average total student budget at a public 2-year university is $14,285 (6). The total cost of becoming an R.N. is then $28,570. If that debt is paid off over 20 years at a 7% interest rate it will end up costing a total of $53,160. At this income, you will be able to deduct student loan interest costs from your federal income taxes (these savings are not included in the calculation below). If you finish nursing school at 20 years old and work until you are 65 years old you will work for 45 years at that median income. We will assume you work 40 hours per week, 50 weeks per year.

$$[(51{,}787 \times 45) - (53{,}160)] \,/\, [(40 \times 50 \times 45) + (3{,}200)\} = \$24.43$$

The adjusted net hourly wage for a registered nurse is $24.43

As of 2009, you would sustain no financial loss if you became a physician instead of a teacher or a nurse. You would, however, sustain a financial loss if you became a physician instead of a dentist. Of course, there are countless other reasons to become a physician, and I hope it is the humanitarian reasons that drive you more than the financial reasons. However, if you are a high school student or college student who is considering becoming a physician, you need to be aware of the financial risk you may take to become a physician. Increasing tuition costs, increasing student loan interest rates, increasing income taxes and decreasing physician reimbursements will only place physicians in a more difficult and deceptive financial situation. Although insurance companies, your government and your patients may expect you to work for free one day, I doubt your student loan lender or your mortgage broker will follow suit to help you out.

Table 5.3. Time Sacrifice by Career

	College (hours)	Medical /Dental School (hours)	Residency (hours)	Hours Training	Years worked after training	Weeks per year	Hours per week	Hours Working	Grand Total (hours)
Nurse (R.N.)*	3,200	-		3,200	45	50	40	90,000	93,200
Teacher	6,400	-	-	6,400	43	38	40	65,360	71,760
Dentist	6,400	11,520	-	17,920	39	45.5	38	67,431	85,351
Physician - Internal Medicine	6,400	15,360	12,000	33,760	36	48	56	96,768	130,528
Physician - General Surgeon	6,400	15,360	20,000	41,760	34	48	60	97,920	139,680

Registered Nurse (R.N.) via the Associates Degree Route

What about scholarships and loan forgiveness programs?

There are many generous scholarships available to college students that can help you minimize your college debt. Unfortunately, the scholarships and grants given to medical students tend to be less generous. There are, however, some government programs that will pay your way through medical school or pay off your medical school debt in return for your services. These programs include the National Health Services Corps, the Indian Health Service, NIH loan repayment programs and the military.

The National Health Service Corps (38)

The National Health Care Service Corps (NHCS) is a government-funded program that rewards physicians for practicing in under-served areas of the United States. You can join this program during medical school or after medical school. If you take the former, scholarship route, the NHCS will pay your medical school tuition directly to your school. This scholarship is limited to four years. You can also join the NHCS after medical school and take advantage of their loan repayment program. This program offers certain specialists $50,000 to help repay their loans in exchange for a 2 year service commitment at an approved NHSC service site. This $50,000 is in addition to what you earn while practicing in these areas. After completing a two year commitment, NHCS physicians may apply for additional commitments and receive additional bonuses to help pay off their loans. Eligible specialties include: Family Medicine, Obstetrics & Gynecology, Internal Medicine, Geriatrics, Pediatrics and Psychiatry. If you go into a specialty not mentioned above, you will not be eligible for this scholarship. Dentists, Family Nurse Practitioners, Nurse Midwives, Physicians' Assistants, Dental Hygienists and certain mental health providers are also eligible. For more information about the National Health Service Corps, go to *nhsc.hrsa.gov/*.

The Indian Health Service (39)

The Indian Health Service is a government-funded program that rewards physicians for practicing on Indian Reservations. This loan repayment program will give physicians up to $20,000 per year in exchange for a two-year service commitment. The Indian Health Service will also pay an additional $4,000 annually to the Internal Revenue Service to offset the increased tax liability from the $20,000 bonus. Many different healthcare providers are eligible. For more information about the Indian Health Service, go to www.loanrepayment.ihs.gov.

National Institutes of Health (NIH) loan repayment programs (LRPs)

Researchers and scientists at universities and nonprofit organizations can apply for extramural LRPs through which the NIH will repay up to $35,000 of student loan debt each year (40). In 2009, 47% of the people who applied for extramural LRPs received them (41). NIH employee researchers can apply for intramural LRPs through which the NIH will repay up to $35,000 of student loan debt each year (40). In 2008, 95% of the people who applied for intramural LRPs received them (42).

To qualify for NIH LRPs (43):

- You must have a doctoral degree from an accredited institution
- Have educational debt equal to or greater than 20% of your base salary
- Be conducting research funded by a domestic nonprofit organization or the U.S. government.
- Spend at least 20 hrs per week conducting this research
- Be a U.S. citizen, U.S. national or permanent resident.

For more information on NIH LRPs, go to *www.LRP.nih.gov*.

The Military

The only medical school run by the military is the Uniformed Services University in Bethesda, Maryland. Students who attend this university must be actively serving in a branch of the military. During medical school they pay no tuition or fees. Moreover, they receive the salary and benefits of an officer throughout medical school (44). After medical school they must enter the military residency match to obtain a residency training position (45). For more information on the military residency match see chapter 16. After their residency training, graduates of the Uniformed Services University have a seven-year active duty service commitment (44). For more information about the Uniformed Services University, go to: *www.usuhs.mil/medschool/somadmissions.html.*

The Army, the Air Force and the Navy have programs that provide financial assistance to college students, medical students and residents. Two commonly utilized programs by medical students and residents are the Health Professions Scholarship Program (HPSP) and the Financial Assistance Program (FAP). Both programs are offered by all three branches of the military.

Health Professions Scholarship Program (HPSP)

- Allopathic and osteopathic medical students at civilian medical schools are eligible
- Tuition, books and most fees are paid for.
- Monthly stipend of $1,992 for up to 48 months
- $20,000 sign-on bonus.
- 45-day active duty training tour during medical school for each year of the scholarship
- You must enter the military residency match
- After you complete residency you are required to serve on active duty for a minimum of 2 years, or the number of years you received the scholarship.

Financial Assistance Program (FAP)

- Available to residents in civilian residency programs
- $45,000 each year
- Monthly stipend of $1,992 in addition to your resident stipend
- 14-day active duty training tour during residency each year the scholarship is awarded
- After you complete residency, you are required serve on active duty for the number of years you received financial assistance plus one extra year.

Contact your local Army, Air Force or Navy Medical Recruiter for more information.

The benefits of joining the military and taking advantage of the HPSP include: less debt, good benefits, guaranteed job when you finish and no malpractice concerns. The sacrifices of joining the military and taking advantage of the HSPS include: less control over residency selection and specialty choice, less freedom to complete fellowships, and less control over location - which can be especially difficult for your spouse or partner.

6   The Decision to Become a Physician

The difficult thing about deciding whether or not to pursue a career as a physician is you that cannot really know what it is like until you are a physician, and becoming one takes a lot of time, effort and money. You can shadow physicians, but you will be unable to appreciate the satisfaction of the patient-physician relationship and the joy of healing people with your knowledge, skills and experience. That satisfaction is experienced near the end of medical school, years after you made the decision to become a physician. Making the decision to become a physician is like religion: you have to have faith that it is the right thing for YOU to do.

If your goal in life is to "help people," there are countless careers that can fulfill that goal. Teachers, nurses, engineers, accountants, chefs, janitors, electricians, mechanics - in reality, any honest job helps people in some way. Hopefully, if you want to be a physician, you have the sincere desire to help people. However, you must also have the desire and discipline to study, work hard, work long hours, be part of a team and spend roughly a decade after college receiving formal education and training. The specialty you go into will determine how intense and how long your residency is, and, for the most part, will determine how hard you will work and study for the rest of your life. Regardless of what you specialize in after medical school, you will be expected to be a "student for life."

Important life decisions with multiple variables are difficult to make. There is no formula or algorithm. Some people try to create an algebraic equation where they quantify how they feel about each factor, quantify the relative importance of each factor, and finally plug the numbers into an equation to produce the answer. This answer is then a number that means what? There is a large degree of error involved with quantifying one's feelings, quantifying relative importance of something and quantifying the yes/no threshold such that the ultimate answer is often useless. The best and only way to make decisions involving multiple variables is to become maximally informed and do what feels right.

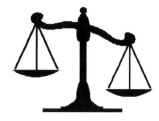

Table 6.1.   *Should I become a physician?*

Sacrifices & Risks	Incentives & Rewards
• Time spent training	• Caring for patients
• Youthful years of your life spent training	• The patient-physician relationship
• Holidays and family events missed	• Improving and saving people's lives
• Working and taking call on nights, weekends and holidays	• Sense of personal accomplishment
• Less time to exercise and eat healthy	• Personal growth
• Less time for hobbies	• A challenging profession
• Delayed childbearing	• Respected profession
• Less time to spend with your children	• Meeting and working with great people
• Inflexible schedule during medical school and residency	• Making friends along the way
• Student loan debt	• Teaching medical students and junior residents
• May not match into the specialty of your choice	• Job security
• Uncertain future physician reimbursements	• Job transferability
• Uncertain future income tax structure	• Potential financial reward

Even after you start medical school, you will have to decide on a day-to-day basis what you are willing to sacrifice to benefit your career. Do you want to get the highest score on the test or do you just want to pass? Should you sleep less so you can study more? Do you have time to exercise? Do you have time to watch the football game with your friends? Do you have time to go shopping with your friends? Every day is an attempt to find that balance. Where you try to find that balance in medical school largely depends on what specialty you want to go into and how competitive it is. Where you try to find that balance during residency depends on what specialty you go into and how intense your training program is. Where you try to find that balance after residency depends on what you want in life.

Are those who became a physician happy with their decision?

In one study, 15,620 practicing physicians in the United States were asked the question, "Thinking very generally about your satisfaction with your overall career in medicine, would you say that you are currently very satisfied, somewhat satisfied, somewhat dissatisfied or very dissatisfied?" Overall, 81% of the physicians working more than 20 hours per week said they were somewhat or very satisfied with their career (46). 18% reported being somewhat or very dissatisfied with their career (47). Among retired physicians, 66% reported being somewhat or very satisfied with their career(46). In another survey of more than 4,700 physicians, 82% reported being somewhat or very satisfied. Pediatricians and specialists reported greater career satisfaction than general internists, family practitioners, psychiatrists and OB-GYNs (48).

Prior to 2008, four out of five practicing physicians in the United States reported being satisfied with their career. This is encouraging, considering the overall U.S. job satisfaction rate is 45% (49, 50).

Does gender affect physician satisfaction?

No. Average physician satisfaction scores do not vary significantly with gender (51). The number of women graduating from medical school each year has been increasing, such that women are now the majority in many medical school classes. In 1999, the results from the Women Physicians' Health Study were published. This survey was completed by 4,501 women physicians, and examined the effect of many variables on career satisfaction. These variables included: specialty, practice type, weekly work hours, call schedule, age, ethnicity, number of children, income and religion. Overall, 84% of women physicians reported that they were "always, almost always or usually satisfied" with their career. 69% of women physicians reported that they would "definitely or probably" become a physician again, with 38% reporting that they would choose a different medical specialty the second time around (52).

Can money buy happiness?

No, but it may be able to buy job satisfaction. The economics literature has shown that, for most jobs, income is the most important predictor of job satisfaction (53). Among physicians, income has been shown to be positively associated with career satisfaction and is often the most statistically significant variable in terms of overall career satisfaction (51). Additionally, income expectations influenced nearly three-fourths of medical students when they decided what to specialize in, as only 26.9% reported that income expectations had no influence on their specialty choice (5).

Isn't taking care of patients satisfying regardless of income?

Yes, taking care of patients is satisfying. However, when physicians are unfairly reimbursed for their services they feel exploited. I think this feeling of exploitation or being taken advantage of is what bothers physicians the most. Compared to physicians in other countries, physicians in the United States have higher incomes. However, fair compensation is relative to the economy in which one lives and works. Physicians invest over 30,000 hours training and spend over a quarter of a million dollars to receive that training. When they finally finish training, they work about 60 hours per week and give over 40% of their income to the government in taxes. They feel exploited because after all that sacrifice they are enslaved to the highly regulated healthcare industry, which pays them unfairly, and there is nowhere else for them to work. They feel most other Americans are being paid fairly and/or receiving tax breaks while they receive neither, and can't even deduct the interest on their student loans from their income taxes. Being taken advantage of or exploited is not satisfying.

Does greater physician satisfaction translate into greater patient satisfaction?

Yes, physician satisfaction has been found to correlate strongly with patient satisfaction (54).

I present the above data to show you that most physicians, as of 2008, were satisfied with their career, especially those physicians with higher incomes. However, I think these statistics are a moot point for someone trying to decide whether or not he/she should become a physician. If I were counseling a crowd of 10,000 pre-medical students, I would feel fairly confident telling them that about 8,000 of them will be satisfied with their decision to become a physician, should the healthcare system not change by the time they are done with training. However, when counseling one person, an individual, YOU - such statistics become a moot point. You need to think about what motivates you, what makes you happy, what fulfills you, what kind of life you want and what sacrifices you are willing to make. Do not think about "80%."

In order to optimize your chances of making the right decision for YOU, you need to become informed by getting exposure to the field of medicine. The personal and confidential aspects of medicine make it quite difficult to get extensive exposure before medical school. The best way to get exposure to the field of medicine in the 21st century is to become part of the healthcare team. Quick ways to become part of this team include going on an international medical mission or getting a job in the U. S. as a nurse's aid, EMT, phlebotomist or patient transporter.

Table 6.2. *When did 2009's first year medical students decide they wanted to be a physician? (4)*

Before High School	19.4 %
During High School or Before College	27.8%
During first 2 yrs of college	24.8%
During junior year of college	12.0 %
During senior year of college	4.0 %
After receiving bachelor's degree	9.9 %
After receiving advanced degree	2.1 %

7   What is a D.O.?

"D.O." stands for "Doctor of Osteopathic Medicine."
"M.D." stands for the Latin "Medicinae Doctor" which means "Doctor of Medicine"

D.O.s are often referred to as "Osteopathic physicians" or "Osteopaths."
M.D.s are referred to as "Allopathic physicians."

D.O.s represent about 6% of the total U.S. physician population (55). However, this minority is growing rapidly considering 21% of U.S. medical students are in osteopathic medical schools.

Similarities:

- Both M.D.s and D.O.s are physicians who may become licensed in all 50 states to prescribe medications and perform surgery.
- Both attend 4 years of medical school.
- Both take the Medical College Admissions Test (MCAT) when applying to medical school.
- Both may take the United States Medical Licensing Exams (USMLE) administered by the National Board of Medical Examiners (NMBE).
- Both apply to allopathic residency programs using the Electronic Residency Application Service (ERAS).
- Both may receive their residency training in ACGME accredited allopathic residency programs.

Differences:

- D.O.s are trained in Osteopathic Manipulative Treatment, or OMT. OMT is the use of stretching, pressure and resistance to treat pain, promote healing and increase mobility (56).
- The American Osteopathic Association (AOA) accredits Osteopathic medical schools (57).

- The Liaison Committee on Medical Education (LCME), which is sponsored by the American Medical Association (AMA) and the Association of American Medical Colleges (AAMC), accredits allopathic medical schools (58).
- Applications to osteopathic medical schools are submitted via the American Association of Colleges of Osteopathic Medicine Application Service (AACOMAS).
- Applications to allopathic medical schools are submitted via the American Medical College Application Service (AMCAS). With the exception of Baylor College of Medicine, all applications to the allopathic and osteopathic medical schools in Texas are submitted via the Texas Medical and Dental Schools Application Service (TMDAS).
- D.O.s are typically required by their institution to take the Comprehensive Osteopathic Medical Licensing Exams (COMLEX); however, they may also take the USMLE if they wish to apply to allopathic residency programs. Similar to the USMLE exams, there are four COMLEX exams: COMLEX Level 1, COMLEX Level 2 CE, COMLEX Level 2PE, and COMLEX Level 3.
- The osteopathic residency match is administered by the National Matching Services (NMS) (59).
- The allopathic residency match is administered by the National Residency Matching Program (NRMP). The allopathic residency match is explained in chapter 16.
- Osteopathic residency programs are accredited by the AOA council on post-doctoral training (60).
- Allopathic residency programs are accredited by the Accreditation Council for Graduate Medical Education (ACGME) (60).
- D.O.s are allowed to train in both osteopathic residency programs (OGME) and allopathic residency programs (ACGME).
- M.D.s are generally not allowed to train in osteopathic residency programs and therefore may only train in allopathic residency programs.

Table 7.1. *Allopathic (M.D.) vs. Osteopathic (D.O.) (8, 10, 11, 61)*

	M.D.	D.O.
Medical School Applicants	42,269	12,617
Medical School Positions	18,390	4,846
Matriculation Rate[11]	43.5%	38.4%
Average MCAT score among accepted applicants	30.8 P	26.19
Average GPA among accepted applicants	3.66	3.49
USMLE Step 1 Pass Rate among first time test takers (62)	94%	81%
USMLE Step 2 CK Pass Rate among first time test takers (62)	96%	87%
USMLE Step 2 CS Pass Rate among first time test takers (62)	97%	87%
USMLE Step 3 Pass Rate (62)	95%	95%

For more information on osteopathic medicine, go to *www.osteopathic.org.*

For a list of AOA accredited osteopathic residency programs, go to : *http://opportunities.osteopathic.org/search.*

For more information on allopathic medicine, go to *www.aamc.org* and *www.ambs.org*

For a list of ACGME accredited allopathic residency programs, go to: *http://www.acgme.org/adspublic.*

---

[11] Matriculation rate refers to the percentage of applicants who started each respective type of medical school. Acceptance rates cannot be calculated because the number of applicants offered acceptance into allopathic medical schools is not known, the number of applicants offered acceptance into osteopathic medical schools is not known and the number of applicants who applied to both allopathic and osteopathic medical schools is not known.

8   The Demographics of Becoming a Physician

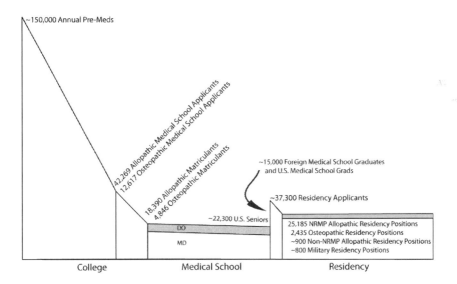

~150,000 Annual Pre-Meds

42,269 Allopathic Medical School Applicants
12,617 Osteopathic Medical School Applicants

18,390 Allopathic Matriculants
4,846 Osteopathic Matriculants

~15,000 Foreign Medical School Graduates and U.S. Medical School Grads

~37,300 Residency Applicants

~22,300 U.S. Seniors

DO

MD

25,185 NRMP Allopathic Residency Positions
2,435 Osteopathic Residency Positions
~900 Non-NRMP Allopathic Residency Positions
~800 Military Residency Positions

College   Medical School   Residency

Over 1.48 million people took the ACT in 2009 (63). 19.3% of ACT test takers planned to go into the health sciences and 27.1% planned to earn a professional degree. 9.3% of ACT test takers plan to go into the health sciences AND earn a professional degree (64).

Over 1.5 million people took the SAT in 2009 (65). 19% of these test-takers plan to major in "Health Professions and Related Clinical Services" and 20% of these test takers plan to obtain a doctoral degree (65). The number of test takers who plan to do both is not available. For purposes of discussion we will assume it is also 9.3%. Probably a little over half of that 9.3% plan to become a physician, say 5% of test takers.

In order to calculate the total number of individuals who took the SAT and/or ACT we need to add the number of ACT and SAT test takers and then subtract the number of people who took both to prevent them from being counted twice. In 2005, 300,437 people took both the SAT and ACT (66) 1.48 million plus 1.5 million minus

0.3 million is 2.95 million individual test takers. 5% of 2.95 million is 147,500. Therefore, there are at about 150,000 annual "pre-meds."

There are 131 accredited allopathic medical schools in the United States (67). U.S. allopathic medical schools received 562,694 applications from 42,269 applicants for the 2009-2010 entering class (8). Of these 42,269 applicants:

- Each applied to an average of 13 allopathic medical schools (8).
- 73% were applying to medical school for the first time (8).
- 52% were men (8).
- 48% were women (8).
- The median age was 23 years old (68).
- 43.5% (18,390) started allopathic medical school in 2009 and were therefore accepted by at least one allopathic medical school (8).
- An unknown number of these applicants were also offered acceptance into osteopathic medical schools and an unknown percentage of them chose to attend an osteopathic medical school.

There are 26 accredited colleges of osteopathic medicine in the United States (69). Osteopathic medical schools received 92,557 applications from 12,617 applicants for the 2009-2010 entering class (11). Of these 12,617 applicants:

- 52% were men (11).
- 48% were women (11).
- 38% (4,846) started osteopathic medical school in 2009 and were therefore accepted by at least one osteopathic medical school (10).
- The median age of both applicants and matriculants was 23 years old (70).
- An unknown number of these applicants were also offered acceptance into allopathic medical schools and an unknown percentage of them chose to attend an allopathic medical school.

96% of people who start medical school will graduate from medical school within 10 yrs (8, 71). The next hurdle, after completing medical school, is being accepted into a residency training program.

In 2009, the National Residency Matching Program (NRMP) represented 4,299 residency training programs offering 25,185 ACGME accredited allopathic training positions (72). Not all allopathic specialties use the NRMP; urology, ophthalmology and pediatric neurology use different matching services. These three specialties represent about 900 additional ACGME accredited allopathic residency training positions. These 26,000 allopathic residency training programs are sought after by U.S. allopathic medical school seniors, U.S. osteopathic medical school seniors, foreign medical school seniors, U.S. medical school graduates and foreign medical school graduates. The residency match takes place each year in March. The majority of residency applicants are senior medical students. In 2009, 93.1% of U.S. allopathic seniors successfully matched into a residency position, with about half matching into their first choice (73). "Medical school graduates" includes those who graduated from medical school prior to the match. This group includes those who took time off between medical school and residency, those who didn't match into a categorical residency program as a senior medical student, those who decided to change specialties and those who decided to change residency programs. Osteopathic residency training positions are only available to osteopathic medical school seniors and graduates. Military residency training positions are only available to those who join the military.

As you can see, there are no guarantees in the process. Less than half of allopathic medical school applicants are accepted and about half of U.S. allopathic medical school seniors match into the residency program of their choice, though most match into the specialty of their choice. For more information on the residency match and the varying competitiveness of different specialties, see chapter 16.

9   Getting Into Medical School

Medical school admissions committees try to predict which applicants are most likely to succeed in medical school and ultimately become excellent physicians. They try to predict this based upon MCAT scores, GPAs, letters of recommendation, previous experiences, personal statements and formal interviews. Which is the most important component of a medical school application is highly debated. However, most would agree that the most important component of one's medical school application is the MCAT score, followed by the GPA, letters of recommendation, career goals, experiences and personality.

The Medical College Admissions Test (MCAT) is a 5 hour and 10 minute standardized exam consisting of 4 sections. The exam is offered from late January through early September each year. You may take the MCAT up to 3 times in one year, but you must register separately for each examination after the scores from your previous examination have been released (74).

The **physical sciences** section is 70 minutes long and contains a total of 52 questions. 13 of these questions are independent or "freestanding," and the other 39 questions follow 7 passages. You will need to rely on your knowledge of general chemistry and physics to solve problems and answer these questions (74).

10 minute break.

The **verbal reasoning** section is 60 minutes long and contains 40 questions. There are 7 passages, each roughly 600 words long, and each passage is followed by 5-7 questions. This section tests your ability to understand, evaluate and apply the information and arguments drawn from each passage. In short, it tests how fast and how accurately you can assimilate what you read. The passages are excerpts from novels, articles or essays. You do not need to, nor can you, study any specific subject matter to prepare for this section. You can, however, develop a strategy for how you read each passage and approach the questions. MCAT preparation courses and books will demonstrate some of these strategies (74).

10 minute break

The **writing sample** section is 60 minutes long. You will write 2 essays. Each essay will stem from a passage or statement that is presented to you. The writing section tests your ability to synthesize concepts and ideas, develop a central idea and present it cohesively and logically. It also evaluates your basic writing skills (74). Two different individuals will independently score each section on a 1 to 6 point scale.[12] Your four scores, two scores from each essay, are added to produce a score between 4 and 24. This numerical "raw" score is then converted to a letter "scaled" score ranging from J to T.

10 minute break

The **biological sciences** section is 70 minutes long and contains a total of 52 questions. You will need to rely on your knowledge of biology and organic chemistry to solve and answer these questions (74).

On the MCAT there is no penalty for guessing, so you do not need to evaluate your confidence level for every answer because you have nothing to lose by guessing. There will be a few questions scattered throughout your exam that are experimental. You are not scored on experimental questions; however, you will not know which questions these are.

The number of questions you answer correctly will determine your raw score. Your raw score is then converted to a scaled score. Some questions are more difficult than others, and different versions of the exam contain different combinations of questions. To compensate for this varying level of difficulty, each question has a conversion factor associated with it that is determined by the number of previous examinees that were able to answer it correctly. Thus, your scaled score is derived from the number of questions you answer correctly and the relative difficulty of those questions (74). Contrary to common belief, the MCAT is not scored from a "normal Gaussian distribution," or bell-curve. MCAT scores, however, tend to naturally distribute themselves into a bell-curve. Therefore, the bell-curve does not create the scores, but rather the scores create the bell-curve.

---

[12]   If the two scores for one essay differ by more than one point, a senior reader will read and score your essay. Scores from senior readers are multiplied by two as only one reader is scoring that essay.

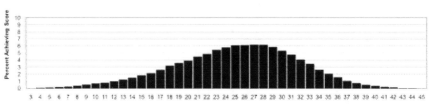

Percentages of MCAT Examinees Achieving Scaled Score Levels and
Associated Percentile Rank Ranges by Area of Assessment
Combined 2009 Administrations N = 79,244

Total Score

Scaled Score	Percent Achieving Score	Percentile Rank Range
45	0.0	99.9—99.9
44	0.0	99.9—99.9
43	0.0	99.9—99.9
42	0.1	99.9—99.9
41	0.2	99.8—99.9
40	0.3	99.5—99.7
39	0.5	99.1—99.4
38	0.7	98.4—99.0
37	1.0	97.4—98.3
36	1.5	95.8—97.3
35	2.0	93.8—95.7
34	2.6	91.2—93.7
33	3.4	87.8—91.1
32	4.0	83.8—87.7
31	4.7	79.1—83.7
30	5.3	73.8—79.0
29	5.8	68.0—73.7
28	6.1	61.9—67.9
27	6.1	55.8—61.8
26	6.1	49.7—55.7
25	6.1	43.7—49.6
24	5.7	38.0—43.6
23	5.4	32.6—37.9
22	4.8	27.8—32.5
21	4.5	23.3—27.7
20	3.9	19.5—23.2
19	3.5	16.0—19.4
18	3.2	12.8—15.9
17	2.6	10.3—12.7
16	2.1	8.2—10.2
15	1.8	6.4—8.1
14	1.5	4.9—6.3
13	1.2	3.7—4.8
12	1.0	2.8—3.6
11	0.8	2.0—2.7
10	0.7	1.3—1.9
9	0.5	0.9—1.2
8	0.3	0.5—0.8
7	0.2	0.3—0.4
6	0.1	0.2—0.2
5	0.1	0.0—0.1
4	0.0	0.0—0.0
3	0.0	0.0—0.0

Scaled Score
Mean   = 25.1
Std Deviation = 6.5

Physical Sciences

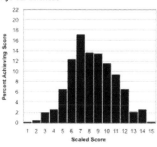

Scaled Score	Percent Achieving Score	Percentile Rank Range
15	0.2	99.9–99.9
14	2.5	97.4–99.8
13	2.1	95.3–97.3
12	6.5	88.8–95.2
11	9.3	79.5–88.7
10	11.5	68.0–79.4
9	13.4	54.6–67.9
8	13.6	41.0–54.5
7	17.1	23.9–40.9
6	12.3	11.6–23.8
5	6.5	5.1–11.5
4	2.5	2.6–5.0
3	2.0	0.6–2.5
2	0.4	0.2–0.5
1	0.1	0.0–0.1

Scaled Score
Mean = 8.3
Std Deviation = 2.5

Verbal Reasoning

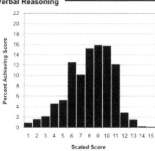

Scaled Score	Percent Achieving Score	Percentile Rank Range
15	0.1	99.9–99.9
14	0.2	99.8–99.9
13	1.5	98.3–99.7
12	2.8	95.5–98.2
11	12.1	83.5–95.4
10	15.7	67.8–83.4
9	15.8	52.0–67.7
8	15.2	36.8–51.9
7	10.1	26.8–36.7
6	12.5	14.2–26.7
5	5.2	9.1–14.1
4	4.6	4.5–9.0
3	2.1	2.5–4.4
2	1.5	0.9–2.4
1	0.8	0.0–0.8

Scaled Score
Mean = 8.1
Std Deviation = 2.5

Writing Sample

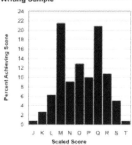

Scaled Score	Percent Achieving Score	Percentile Rank Range
T	0.7	99.4–99.9
S	5.0	94.4–99.3
R	10.7	83.8–94.3
Q	20.8	62.9–83.7
P	9.9	53.0–62.8
O	12.8	40.2–52.9
N	9.0	31.1–40.1
M	21.4	9.7–31.0
L	6.2	3.4–9.6
K	2.6	0.8–3.3
J	0.7	0.0–0.7

Scaled Score
75th Percentile = Q
50th Percentile = O
25th Percentile = M

Biological Sciences

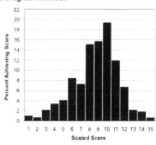

Scaled Score	Percent Achieving Score	Percentile Rank Range
15	0.6	99.5–99.9
14	1.8	97.7–99.4
13	2.1	95.6–97.6
12	6.6	88.9–95.5
11	11.9	77.1–88.8
10	19.4	57.7–77.0
9	15.7	42.0–57.6
8	15.1	26.8–41.9
7	7.2	19.5–26.7
6	8.4	11.2–19.5
5	4.0	7.2–11.1
4	3.3	3.9–7.1
3	2.1	1.7–3.8
2	0.7	1.1–1.6
1	1.0	0.0–1.0

Scaled Score
Mean = 8.7
Std Deviation = 2.6

Table 9.1.   *Average MCAT Score and GPA of U.S. Allopathic Applicants vs. Matriculants (61)*

	Applicants	Matriculants
MCAT Verbal Reasoning	9.0	9.8
MCAT Physical Sciences	9.2	10.3
MCAT Biological Sciences	9.8	10.8
MCAT Writing Section	O	P
MCAT Total/Composite	27.9 O	30.8 P
GPA – Science	3.41	3.60
GPA – Non-science	3.64	3.74
GPA Total	3.51	3.66

Table 9.2.   *Average MCAT Score and GPA of Osteopathic Applicants vs. Matriculants (10, 11)*

	Applicants	Matriculants
MCAT Verbal Reasoning	8.38	8.59
MCAT Physical Sciences	8.18	8.38
MCAT Biological Sciences	8.93	9.22
MCAT Writing Section	O	O
MCAT Total/Composite	25.5 O	26.19 O
GPA – Science	3.31	3.41
GPA – Non-science	3.53	3.59
GPA Total	3.42	3.49

Why do medical school admission committees place so much weight on MCAT scores?

An applicant's MCAT score is the only standardized piece of objective data that admissions committees have to compare applicants to one another. Moreover, multiple studies have shown a strong correlation between an applicant's MCAT score and their performance in medical school and on licensing exams (12, 75-78). Undergraduate GPAs have also been shown to correlate with performance in medical school and on medical licensing exams; however, MCAT scores have consistently shown to be a better predictor of performance than undergraduate GPAs (75, 78). Performance in osteopathic medical school and on the COMLEX exams was also predicted by both undergraduate GPA and MCAT scores with undergraduate GPA being a better predictor than MCAT scores (79).

What should you do if you do poorly on the MCAT?

Take it again. 35% of matriculating U.S. allopathic medical students in 2009 reported taking the MCAT more than once (4).

Performance on undergraduate and graduate coursework as evidenced by one's GPA is also important. The problem with using GPAs to compare applicants is that medical school applicants come from different institutions with different majors. Admissions committees do their best to determine if an applicant's GPA represents academic achievement. They consider the institution, the major, the number of classes taken each semester, trends in GPA, other responsibilities while in college, and so on.

Ultimately, clinical performance and overall performance as a physician is most highly correlated with personal characteristics such as motivation, conscientiousness, integrity, empathy and a robust psychological constitution (80). One could argue that doing well on standardized exams takes motivation, a robust psychological constitution and a good work ethic, and therefore performance on standardized exams may very well correlate with some of these admirable personal characteristics. Of course, doing well on the MCAT does not necessarily mean you are a good person. Everyone knows an individual of questionable moral character who scored really high on the MCAT, and, hopefully, other components of the application process will identify these applicants. However, you have to admit that, on average, people who do well on the MCAT are probably more likely to succeed in medical school and as a physician than people who do poorly. Should medical schools prefer applicants who do poorly on the MCAT? Of course not. Try not to think of standardized exams as a burden; rather, think of them as an opportunity to distinguish yourself.

Because it takes about a decade to train a physician, medical schools typically prefer to train younger people. A 23 year-old will be finished when they are about 33 years old and will likely be able to serve society as a physician for at least 30 years. A 35 year-old will not be finished until they are about 45 and will be able to spend significantly less time serving society as a physician. Additionally, age has been shown to have an inverse correlation with USMLE Step 2 performance, with older medical students having lower scores than their younger classmates (12). Medical students often joke that older, or "non-traditional," medical students don't do quite as well, on average, because they know how good life can be and tend to have more interests outside medical school, while younger, "traditional," medical students don't know what life is like outside academia and thus remain more focused due to their ignorance.

Should you double major?

No, not if your only reason for double majoring is because you think it will help you get into medical school. Your time and effort would be more effective if directed towards studying for the MCAT, maintaining a solid GPA, doing some research, working as an EMT, and so on.

Should you get an extra degree or master's degree?

No, not if your only reason for doing so is because you think it will help you get into medical school. Apply and try to start medical school as soon as possible. Prolonging the process and increasing your debt load is only worth it if you were not accepted to medical school and you need something productive to do with your time before you reapply. If your undergraduate academic performance is below par, you can use graduate studies as an opportunity to show academic achievement and a change in attitude. However, doing well for one year of graduate school will probably not look better than an applicant who performed well academically their entire college career. Applicants who consistently perform well academically are often assumed to have a more robust psychological constitution than applicants whose performance fluctuates.

Will having a master's degree help you get into residency?

Probably not. Among U.S. allopathic seniors, 11.0% of those who successfully matched into the specialty of their choice had a graduate degree while 13.6% of those who did not match into the specialty of their choice had a graduate degree (28).

Should you do research?

Yes, if you can do it without prolonging the process or compromising your MCAT score and/or your GPA. Professors and physicians in academia regard research highly. In the world of academia, one of the considerations for faculty promotion is research productivity. How many articles have they published recently? In which journals? How much money are they bringing to the institution via research grants? Research is important for the careers of faculty and it is important for the future of medicine. The people who will be reviewing your application and interviewing you will be these faculty members. So, even if you hate pipettes and p-values, you should try to get involved with some type of research.

Table 9.3. *Matriculating U.S. Allopathic Medical Students (4)*

Volunteered or worked in the healthcare field	93.3 %
MCAT preparation course	67.9 %
Laboratory research in college	57.0 %
Non-degree post-baccalaureate program to complete premedical requirements	8.3 %

Should you take time off between college and medical school?

It depends on why you are taking a year off. If you want to live life a little and travel the world, go for it! If you want to work off some of your college debt or save up for medical school, you better have some serious earning power to justify taking a year off, because you are simply delaying your ability to work as a physician by one year. Some foreign medical schools and osteopathic medical schools charge an excessive amount for tuition. What they are doing is exploiting desperate pre-meds who were not accepted by other medical schools. Delaying your medical education in an effort to attend a more affordable medical school may actually cost less in the end. 46.4% of the 2009 matriculating U.S. allopathic medical school class reported that at least one year had passed since they graduated from college. 86.6% worked during this time, and 67.2% continued taking courses of some type (4).

Should you apply to M.D.- PhD programs?

Yes, if you want to earn both an M.D. and a PhD. These programs tend to be more competitive than traditional M.D. programs, so don't apply to these programs in an effort to increase your chances of being accepted to medical school. M.D.- PhD programs are typically structured such that M.D.- PhD students leave their medical school class after the basic science years to complete their PhD, which takes about 4 additional years. They then return to finish their 3rd and 4th years of medical school after finishing their PhD. For the 2009 incoming class, 1,703 people applied for M.D. - PhD. positions, 816 were accepted and 601 matriculated (81). The mean MCAT score and GPA among those who matriculated into M.D.-PhD programs was 34.3 and 3.74, respectively (82). Does earning a PhD help you land a residency position? Yes, it makes you a more competitive applicant, but not enough to justify doing it for that reason. In 2009, 4.2% of successfully matched U.S. Seniors had a Ph.D., while 3.9% of U.S. Seniors who didn't match had a Ph.D. (28).

You weren't accepted into medical school, now what?

If you want to be a physician, improve your application and apply again. Meet with a pre-med advisor or medical school dean and figure out what the weakest and most improvable parts of your application are. If your GPA is 3.0 and your MCAT score is 25, you should focus on bringing up your MCAT score. It will take a long time to move a 3.0 GPA after 4 years, as a 3.0 GPA earned over 4 years will only become a 3.2 GPA if you earn a 4.0 GPA your fifth year. Your MCAT score is earned over 5 hours and 10 minutes and is not pulled down by any previous score. Each time is a new opportunity. Moreover, as explained above, the MCAT has been shown to be a more useful predictor of success in allopathic medical school than your undergraduate GPA.

In 2009, only 29% of matriculating allopathic medical students said they would pursue training in dentistry, osteopathic medicine, veterinary medicine, nursing, physician's assistant or chiropractic in the event that they were not accepted to a U.S. allopathic medical school (4). Keep in mind that this group is also notoriously uninformed, as about half of them didn't know what being board certified meant, even after they started medical school. Furthermore, at least a third of my MD colleagues have mentioned that if they could do it all over again, they would choose to become a dentist, physician's assistant, nurse practitioner, nurse anesthetist or perfusionist – instead of becoming a physician.

Some medical schools have masters degree programs that "funnel" students into their medical school. They are usually pharmacology or physiology masters degree programs. Be skeptical of these programs. They are often very expensive and may not actually help you. Find out what the track record of their students is: How many of them are ultimately accepted into medical school? How many of them would have been accepted without entering this master's degree program? What is the added benefit?

You think you should complete more coursework, what should you study?

There is no right answer to this question. However, knowledge of biostatistics can make you very valuable to future faculty mentors, department chairmen, residency program directors, etc. Remember, research is important for their careers, so if you are a statistics wizard you can help them with their research and hopefully they will help you.

Should you go to an allopathic medical school or an osteopathic medical school?

If you are interested in osteopathic manipulative treatment, naturopathic treatments and a more holistic approach – you may fit in best at an osteopathic school. If you think you may want to go into one of the allopathic specialties that tend to accept few osteopathic applicants, then you may be better served attending an allopathic medical school. For more information on the success of osteopathic applicants in the allopathic residency match, see table 16.2.

You weren't accepted into an allopathic medical school. Should you go to an osteopathic medical school or wait one year and re-apply to allopathic medical schools?

Going to an osteopathic medical school will not close the door on any future opportunities per se. Osteopathic medical school graduates can attend both allopathic and osteopathic residency programs, while allopathic medical school graduates can only attend allopathic residency programs. Some of the more competitive allopathic specialties accept few osteopathic medical school seniors and grads (see table 16.2 for more information on the residency match). Is this because they discriminate against osteopaths? Probably not. Competitive specialties have the luxury of being more selective in choosing their residents, so they are naturally going to choose the best, most competitive applicants, who more often come from allopathic medical schools. This is not because osteopathic medical schools do a poor job training their students. It is because, on average, matriculants of allopathic medical schools tend to be more competitive to begin with as they have higher MCAT scores, GPAs, etc. So, if you are accepted by an osteopathic medical school, but no allopathic medical schools, and you think you may want to go into a competitive allopathic specialty, you have to realistically ask yourself if it is worth forgoing the opportunity to attend an osteopathic medical school in hopes that you will be accepted to an allopathic medical school next year. Why will you be a better applicant to allopathic medical schools next year? If you are accepted to an allopathic medical school, do you have what it takes to be a competitive allopathic applicant at the end of medical school, despite not being a competitive enough applicant to be accepted by an allopathic medical school the first time around? In other words, will forgoing the opportunity to attend an osteopathic medical school in the hopes of attending an allopathic medical school really help you in the end? If you do decide to wait one year and reapply to allopathic medical schools next year, you should definitely reapply to osteopathic medical schools the following year as well.

You weren't accepted into an allopathic medical school - should you go to a foreign medical school or wait one year and re-apply to allopathic medical schools?

Going to a foreign medical school will not close the door on any future opportunities per se. Some of the more competitive allopathic specialties accept a few foreign medical school seniors and grads (see table 16.2 for more information on the residency match).

Table 9.4.   *Allopathic Residency Match Rates(73)*

Applicants	36,972
Training Positions	25,185
Overall Match Rate	71.4%
U.S. Allopathic Medical School Senior Match Rate	93.1%
Osteopathic Medical School Seniors and Graduates Match Rate	69.9%
U.S. citizen Foreign Medical School Graduate Match Rate	47.8%
U.S. Allopathic Medical School Graduate Match Rate	44.6%
Non-U.S. Citizen Foreign Medical School Graduate Match Rate	41.6%
All Others	60.5%

Why is the match rate among U.S. allopathic medical school graduates so much lower than the match rate among U.S. allopathic medical school seniors?

The vast majority of people match into a residency position in March of their senior year of medical school and start residency July 1st after they have graduated from medical school, so they match into residency as a medical student but start residency as a medical school graduate. The match rate among U.S. allopathic medical school graduates is lower because that population includes people who didn't match when they were a senior medical student and are trying again after they graduated. This group also includes people who want to change residency programs and/or specialties.

Self-Appraisal

The most important thing you need to do when you are faced with rejection and disappointment is to maintain a healthy self-appraisal.

Self-appraisal refers to how one evaluates their own successes and failures on a day-to-day basis. Let's say you don't do as well on a test as you would have liked to. Is your poor performance due to the weather that day, the seat you sat in, what you had for breakfast, the professor's poor teaching, the test itself, your not studying enough, your not studying efficiently or poor time management? Those people with healthy self-appraisal will look to themselves first, attributing their shortcomings to their own decisions and actions.

Below are some common statements I have heard though the years from pre-medical students and medical students, which illustrate poor self-appraisal.

"I don't need to study."

As per a literature search performed on June 14, 2009, there have been no reported cases of infants being born with an understanding of renal physiology or the ability to perform a pancreatoduodenectomy. You are, however, born with an ability to learn. Some people are able to learn things more quickly than others; however, that innate ability is beyond anyone's control. Next time you see a group of students in the library holding a discussion about how gifted they are intellectually, remind yourself that it is no different than a group of students in the library holding a discussion about the color of their eyes. What a waste of time! What you do have control over is how much, how intensely and how effectively you study. So, yes, you need to study – everyone needs to study.

"Oh no! I didn't study at all for this test."

No one should ever be ashamed of doing his or her best and failing. Those who should be ashamed are those who don't do their best for fear of failure. It is hard on one's self esteem to put a lot of effort into something and then fail. On the other hand, if one puts forth little effort and then fails, one can always tell oneself, "I could have done better *if* I had put forth more effort," which is much easier on one's self-esteem. However, making less than optimal effort to protect your self-esteem will prevent you from reaching your potential and may be detrimental to your success.

"Grades don't matter." "Exams don't matter."

The purpose of "grades" and "exams" is to evaluate your fund of knowledge and performance. Your patients and your career will both be better served if you know what you are doing and can perform well clinically. If you do poorly on an exam or in a class, figure out why you performed sub-optimally and learn from it.

"I am just a bad test taker."

That may be true and it is both unfortunate and unfair. However, I have found that most students who claim to be "bad test takers" are actually "poorly prepared test takers." When I tutor students, I like to teach them test-taking strategy by going over their exams with them. Most students simply did not understand the information but incorrectly blamed their poor performance on some factor that is out of their control. In an untimed environment, with me walking them through the question one-on-one, I could tell it wasn't that they were "tricked by the test," but rather that they didn't understand the material because they didn't study enough. There were a few students who did actually understand the material, yet still did poorly on the exam. These students choked. They choked because they weren't confident in their understanding of the material, and spent too much time second-guessing their answers and stressing out about the importance of the exam. If you are a "bad test taker," think of it as an adversity you must overcome by being extra-prepared for your exams. Being extra-prepared will give you a better understanding of the material on the test and more confidence in your understanding of the material. Being well prepared by thoroughly understanding the material is the best long-term treatment for "bad test takers." You cannot expect society or your future patients to make an exception for you and accept unsatisfactory performance.

"I don't need to know this."

If you are a high school student or college student, you probably don't know what you need to know and what you don't. You cannot yet appreciate that an understanding of fluid dynamics in physics class is necessary to understand the physiology of the circulatory system, that an understanding of general chemistry is necessary to understand renal physiology, and that an understanding of Ohms law is necessary to understand neurophysiology.

Healthy self-appraisal is much more difficult and painful than blaming your failures on external factors. Over the course of your life you will be much more successful if you learn from your failures and gain an appreciation for your strengths and your weaknesses.

Stay focused, work hard, develop and maintain a healthy self-appraisal and don't let your drive for perfection take the joy out of life.

10   Choosing a Medical School

To maximize your chances of being offered acceptance, you should apply to a number of different medical schools of varying levels of competitiveness. You should also apply to all the medical schools in whichever state you are a legal resident, as many medical schools have a preference for students from their state.

If you are fortunate enough to be accepted to more than one medical school and are faced with the decision of which school to attend, here are some things to think about.

1.   Location

Living near family and friends has its advantages. Living somewhere you want to live is also nice, as medical school will account for at least 4 years, which is about 7% of your remaining life.

2.   Reputation

In your fourth year of medical school you will be applying for residency training positions. Your academic record will be interpreted in the context of where it is from. If you work hard at any U.S. allopathic medical school you can become a competitive applicant for any residency program. Attending a higher profile medical school with a good reputation, however, does have some advantages, such as more research opportunities and more well-known faculty members who can write letters of recommendation.

3.   Cost

As explained in chapter 5, student debt proliferates until you are done with residency and can start paying it off with your post-tax income. You can minimize this burden by attending a more affordable medical school. Do not be mislead by your first year financial aid package: many of those "scholarships" and "grants" may not be promised to you for every year.

4. Faculty

When you apply to residency you will need to have letters of recommendation from faculty in that field. The most persuasive letter of recommendation comes from a nationally known and respected leader in that specialty who knows you well. Some studies have shown that "what a letter of recommendation says" about an applicant is nearly as important as "who says it" (83). If you don't attend an institution with well-known faculty in the specialty you want to go into, you can do rotations at other institutions with well-known faculty in that specialty. These "away rotations" are typically done at the beginning of your fourth year of medical school.

5. Research opportunities

If you want to go into a competitive specialty, you should try to do some research in that field. As explained in chapter 9, research is one of the ways faculty are evaluated and promoted. Residency programs like applicants who have done some research in medical school because they hope it will translate into research during residency, which will benefit them.

6. Grading System

Some medical schools have no grades, and students simply pass or fail. Pass/Fail grading systems tend to create a non-competitive atmosphere. This may seem like a nice feature; however, it will result in residency programs having less data about your performance in medical school, so they will rely more heavily upon USMLE scores, etc. Some medical schools award grades based on a bell-curve, with the top 20% of scores being given an A, the next 30% a B, etc. These medical schools tend to have a more competitive atmosphere, but this could give you an opportunity to distinguish yourself.

7. Class Size

The class size of a medical school is typically limited by the 3rd and 4th year clinical clerkships. The more clinical services an institution has or is affiliated with, the more learning opportunities they have for 3rd and 4th year medical students and the more 1st year students they can admit. Regardless of how many students are sitting in the lecture hall with you during your 1st and 2nd years, there will probably only be one to three medical students on a clinical service during your 3rd and 4th years. Say you are on your 3rd year pediatrics rotation; your clinical service, or team, will probably be comprised of an attending physician, an upper level resident, two interns and two medical students. There may be more medical students on the pediatrics clerkship at that time, but they will be on other teams. Class size is really only noticed during the first two years of medical school. After that you will probably be with a couple other medical students on any given clinical service.

8. Curriculum

There are many different ways medical schools teach the basic sciences. Some teach by subject, e.g. pathology, microbiology, pharmacology, etc. Some teach by organ system, where the pathology, microbiology, pharmacology, physical exam, etc. for the pulmonary system is taught together or integrated. Medical schools incorporate a variable amount of problem-based learning (PBL). PBL is the use of clinical cases to teach the basic sciences. A 67-year-old male with a past medical history of chronic obstructive pulmonary disease (COPD) presents to the emergency department with a 3 day history of fevers, dyspnea and cough productive of purulent sputum. You would then study COPD, chest x-rays, microbes that cause COPD exacerbations, medications used to treat COPD exacerbations, etc. pertaining to this case.

The 3rd and 4th year curriculum will vary among medical schools with regard to when clinical clerkships start, where they take place and how much time you have for elective rotations.

Some medical schools start the clinical clerkships in July, two years after you start medical school. Some medical schools start the clinical clerkships earlier, one-and-a-half years after you start medical school. When they start the clinical clerkships depends on how much time they dedicate to the basic sciences. Where you do your clinical rotations depends on the clinical services your medical school is affiliated with. If your medical school is affiliated with an underfunded, resident-run county hospital you will likely have multiple rotations there. As a medical student you will likely be given more responsibility and allowed to "do more" at a resident run county hospital than at an erudite, private, tertiary care center.

9. Seeing patients in the First Year

Many medical schools try to sell their institution to applicants by touting patient interaction as a first-year medical student. Interacting with patients as a first year medical student isn't necessarily a bad thing, but you shouldn't let this influence your decision. Just because you have been in medical school for 3 months and they gave you a white coat doesn't mean you have any idea what you are doing. Interacting with patients is great, and I hope you are able to do so in college as an EMT or a nurse's aide. But interacting with patients in your first year of medical school as a "doctor" is awkward and no more valuable than when you interacted with them in college – after all, you were in college just a few months ago.

10. Mission of the Institution

You should try to attend an institution whose goals and missions align with yours. If you want to be a family physician, attend an institution that strives to produce primary care physicians. If you want to be a researcher, attend an institution that strives to produce physician-scientists. If you want to be a pediatric heart transplant surgeon, attend an institution that produces specialists and has a good surgery department.

11. Success in the Residency Match

You want to attend a medical school that will maximize your chance of success in the residency match, as that is the next hurdle in your medical education. Unfortunately, there is no great marker of how successful a medical school's seniors are in the match. If the medical school does the right thing and encourages their students to shoot for the stars and rank highly competitive residency programs as their #1 choice, then the percentage of their graduates matching into their first choice will be lower than if the school discouraged their students from aiming high. What you can look at to get an idea of a medical school's success in the match is the percentage of students matching into the specialty of their choice and the specialties their students go into. If the majority of a medical school's students match into the specialty of their choice and a good number of their students go into competitive specialties – then you can assume the medical school does a pretty good job making their students competitive residency applicants. For more information on the residency match, see chapter 16.

Regardless of where you go, you will probably be satisfied with your medical education. 86.6% of graduating allopathic medical students in 2009 either agreed or strongly agreed with the statement, "Overall, I am satisfied with the quality of my medical education" (5).

Medical School Admission Requirements (MSAR) published by the AAMC© contains valuable information about each U.S. allopathic medical school: *http://www.aamc.org/students/applying/msar.htm*

11   Medical School Application

Medical school admissions committees put all the components of your application into a "relative context." They then try to figure out if you would be a good physician and decide if you would fit in at their institution. What I mean by "relative context" is the timbre of your application when all components are considered. If you took only a couple classes each semester to make sure you would earn straight A's, yet did nothing else with your time – they won't be impressed. If you only took a couple of classes each semester; but worked full-time, raised 4 children, coached a soccer team and earned straight A's – they might be impressed. On the same note, they will probably be more impressed by a "B" in organic chemistry at Harvard than an "A" in organic chemistry at a community college. They consider everything relative to its context, and do their best to figure out what kind of person you are and what you are capable of.

You will apply to most U.S. Medical Schools online via the American Medical College Application Service (AMCAS).

AMCAS application sections (84):

1.   Identifying Information

- Legal name, Preferred name, Alternate names
- Identification numbers such as your social security number or social insurance number
- Birth date, Birth location
- Gender

2.   Schools Attended

- High school from which you graduated
- Colleges
    - List every post-secondary institution where you have been enrolled for at least one course. List them even if credits were transferred, not earned or you withdrew.
    - List all degrees earned or you are expected to earn

    o   List all majors and minors

3. Biographic Information

- Citizenship, Legal Residence
- Languages Spoken
- Ethnicity, Race
- Parent/Guardian demographics
- Sibling demographics
- Felony information

4. Course Work

- List the course name, course number, credits earned and grade received for every course you have been enrolled in at any U.S. or Canadian post-secondary institution. The only transfer grades and credits that will be accepted are from official study-abroad coursework taken outside the U.S. and Canada. If you took a course at a U.S. institution which was transferred to another U.S. institution, the transferred credits will not be counted. You must enter the coursework as a separate entry for the institution that granted you the credit originally.
- Your official transcripts will be reviewed by AMCAS to verify that the grades you entered are accurate.
- AMCAS will then calculate your GPA based on their scale.
  - All grades and credit hours are included in your calculated GPA regardless of whether or not they count toward a degree.
  - All attempts of repeated coursework will be counted separately.
  - All grades and credit hours of failed coursework will be included in your calculated GPA.
  - Post-baccalaureate coursework is included in your undergraduate GPA; however, it is also calculated separately and reported as your "post-baccalaureate GPA."
  - Pass/Fail, AP and CLEP coursework is not included in the GPA calculation.
  - The following designations will not affect your GPA because no grades will be entered for:
    - Audited courses
    - Current coursework
    - Exempted coursework
    - "No record" or NR coursework as a result of school error
    - Courses from which you withdrew

5. Work / Activities

- Up to 15 experiences may be entered
- Experience type:
    - Employment experiences
    - Extracurricular activities
    - Awards, Honors
    - Publications
    - Research experiences
    - Volunteer experiences
- Experience name
- Experience dates and time spent each week
- Organization name and contact information
- Description of up to 1,325 characters

6. Letters of Evaluation

- Up to 10 letters of evaluation may be associated with your application. 1 individual letter, 1 committee letter and 1 letter packet are each equivalent to one letter. Most medical schools will only accept 3 to 4 letters. The purpose of being able to associate 10 letters with your application allows you to target specific medical schools with specific letters, should you wish to do that.
- You must enter the contact information of each letter writer.

7. Medical Schools

- Designate the medical schools to which you want to submit an application.
- Designate the letters of recommendation you want each school to receive. The number required and the maximum number allowed varies by school.

8. Personal Statement

- Your personal essay explaining why you selected the field of medicine, what motivates you and any other information about yourself you would like to discuss such as challenges, hardships or fluctuations in your academic record. Your personal statement may be up to 5300 characters in length.
- MD/PhD applicants will need to write and upload two additional essays
    - MD/PhD essay explaining why you want to earn an MD and a PhD (3000 character maximum).
    - Significant research experience essay (10,000 character maximum).

9. Standardized Tests

- All MCAT scores will be automatically uploaded to your AMCAS application.
- AMCAS does not want your SAT or ACT scores. Some secondary applications may give you the option of disclosing these scores.
- AMCAS gives you the option to upload GRE, LSAT and GMAT scores. Unless you are applying to an MD/MBA or MD/JD program, some schools may find it strange that you took the LSAT and/or GMAT, so be sure to explain this in your personal statement if you choose to upload these scores.

For more information about the American Medical College Application Service (AMCAS) go to *http://www.aamc.org/students/amcas/start.htm*

Medical schools in Texas use the Texas Medical and Dental School Application Service (TMDSAS) instead of AMCAS. Exceptions to this include Baylor College of Medicine and all MD/PhD programs, which use AMCAS. Texas medical schools have a matching process through which applicants are offered admission. More information on TMDSAS and the admission matching process can be found at:
http://www.utsystem.edu/tmdsas/homepage.html.

Application deadlines vary by medical school. It is usually best to submit your application as early as possible. Remember that after you complete and submit your AMCAS and TMDSAS applications it will take some time for these organizations to receive all the components of your application, process it and send it out to the medical schools.

12   Life in Medical School

The **first and second years** of medical school are spent primarily in the classroom and the library studying the basic sciences. Subjects covered include:

Anatomy, Biochemistry, Molecular Biology, Cell Biology, Genetics, Histology, Physiology, Neuroscience, Neuroanatomy, Human Behavior, Pathophysiology, Pathology, Microbiology, Pharmacology, Physical Examination, Biostatistics, Epidemiology, Nutrition, Immunology, Clinical Medicine and Ethics.

Some medical schools have condensed the traditional two-years of basic science into less than two years, which leaves their students with more time for the required clinical clerkships and elective rotations.

Step 1 of the United States Medical Licensing Exam (USMLE) is usually taken after finishing your basic science coursework, which places it at or near the end of your second year of medical school. USMLE Step 1 is an eight-hour, computerized exam consisting of 336 questions. There are seven sections, each containing 48 questions. Examinees are given 60 minutes for each section and 60 minutes of total break time, rationed at the examinees' discretion throughout the day. If an examinee finishes a section early, the extra time is added to their break time. Step 1 is administered at Prometric™ testing centers throughout the world. U.S. medical students register to take the exam through the National Board of Medical Examiners (NBME), and International medical students and graduates register to take the exam through the Educational Commission for Foreign Medical Graduates (ECFMG). The exam covers anatomy, biochemistry, nutrition, histology, physiology, neuroscience, neuroanatomy, behavioral science, genetics, pathology, microbiology, pharmacology, molecular biology, immunology, biostatistics and medical ethics. It currently costs $505 to take the exam (85). *Once you pass the exam, you cannot take it again in an effort to achieve a higher score.* That being said, if you want to get into a competitive residency program, you should not take the exam until you are well prepared. The best way to prepare for Step 1 is to do well in the basic sciences during your first and second years of medical school. Most students also allocate one to two months to prepare for the exam.

The National Board of Medical Examiners (NBME) discontinued the percentile scoring system about a decade ago. Step 1 examinees are now given a three-digit score and a two-digit score. The two-digit score is calculated from the three-digit score such that a passing score, 188, is equal to 75 (86). Most residency programs use the three digit score, as it is more specific. The NBME no longer releases the percentile for each score. In "Charting Outcomes in the Match," the National Residency Matching Program (NRMP) stated the mean USMLE Step 1 score of U.S. senior applicants and independent applicants, as well as the standard deviation of these scores (28). A step 1 score was reported for 92.9% of residency applicants (28). I calculated the "overall" mean step 1 score and standard deviation from the number of each type of applicant, and the respective mean score and standard deviation.[13] Given the overall mean step 1 score and standard deviation, and assuming the scores distribute themselves into a normal "Gaussian" distribution, I was able to calculate the "assumed" percentile of each score. These are not the actual percentiles; however, they can give you an idea as to what a "competitive" Step 1 score is.

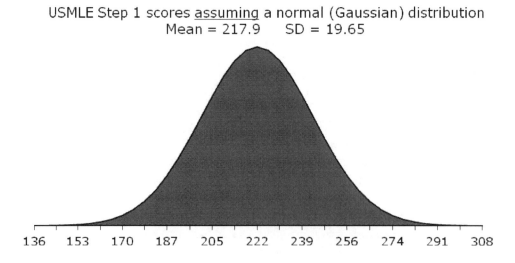

USMLE Step 1 scores <u>assuming</u> a normal (Gaussian) distribution
Mean = 217.9   SD = 19.65

| 136 | 153 | 170 | 187 | 205 | 222 | 239 | 256 | 274 | 291 | 308 |

---

[13]   Among U.S. Seniors, the mean USMLE Step 1 score was 224.3 and the standard deviation was 19.6. Among independent applicants, the mean USMLE Step 1 score was 211 and the standard deviation was 19.7.
[(224.3 x 14958) + (211.0 x 13759)] / (14958 + 13759) = 217.9
[(19.6 x 14958) + (19.7 x 13759)] / (14958 + 13759) = 19.65

Table 12.1. *USMLE Step 1 Score Percentiles assuming a normal (Gaussian) distribution*
Mean = 217.9 SD = 19.65

Score	Percentile	Score	Percentile	Score	Percentile	Score	Percentile
<172	1	205	26	218	51	232	76
176	2	206	27	219	52	232	77
181	3	207	28	219	53	233	78
184	4	207	29	220	54	234	79
186	5	208	30	220	55	234	80
187	6	208	31	221	56	235	81
189	7	209	32	221	57	236	82
190	8	209	33	222	58	237	83
192	9	210	34	222	59	237	84
193	10	210	35	223	60	238	85
194	11	211	36	223	61	239	86
195	12	211	37	224	62	240	87
196	13	212	38	224	63	241	88
197	14	212	39	225	64	242	89
198	15	213	40	226	65	243	90
198	16	213	41	226	66	244	91
199	17	214	42	226	67	245	92
200	18	214	43	227	68	247	93
201	19	215	44	228	69	248	94
201	20	215	45	228	70	250	95
202	21	216	46	229	71	252	96
203	22	216	47	229	72	255	97
203	23	217	48	230	73	258	98
204	24	217	49	230	74	>264	99
205	25	217.9	50	231	75		

The **third and fourth years** of medical school consist of clinical clerkships in various specialties. After 4 years of college and 2 years of medical school, you finally enter the clinical realm. This requires a change in perspective. For 6 years you have been, for the most part, studying and learning independently. Even if you studied in groups, the success of your study-mates didn't depend on your success, and your success didn't depend on the success of your study-mates. Once you enter the clinical realm, you will become part of a team and your patient's success will depend on the team's, not an individual's, performance. No physicians work alone. Even radiologists and pathologists have techs, secretaries and administrators who they must work with.

Required clerkships include Internal Medicine, Surgery, Pediatrics, Obstetrics & Gynecology, Psychiatry, Family Medicine and Neurology. The order in which you take your required clinical clerkships and how much time you have to do elective rotations varies among medical schools.

The most important decision you will make during medical school is what you will specialize in. What will all this training and student loan debt culminate in? What will you do for the rest of your career? What you decide to specialize in will determine how you arrange your fourth year schedule and which residency programs you will apply to in September of your fourth year. This decision may sneak up on you. By the time you finish your required clinical clerkships there is little time left to figure out what area of medicine interests you most and what kind of practice you want.

In order to get the letters of recommendation you need, you may have to schedule certain rotations with specific faculty members. Therefore, you will need to know what you want to specialize in prior to making your fourth year schedule. Because you need to figure out what you want to specialize in by the end of your third year of medical school, I encourage you to go exploring during your required clinical clerkships. If you are on internal medicine and you order a peripheral blood smear on one of your patients, go down to pathology and look at it with the pathologists. If you order a CT scan on a patient, go down to radiology and look at it with one of the radiologists. When you are on surgery, go into as many different operations as you can. While in the operating room, help the anesthesiologist so you can see what they do. If one of your patients is going to the endoscopy suite for an esophagogastroduodenoscopy, go with them and see what the gastroenterologists do. When you are on spring break, make arrangements to spend the day with physicians in specialties you want to learn more about.

In order to increase their chances of matching at a particular residency program, some fourth year medical students go to other institutions to complete rotations. These are often referred to as "away rotations." Most commonly, the students who do "away rotations" are those who are applying to competitive specialties. Doing rotations at other institutions gives you an opportunity to see what a program is like and gives the residents and faculty at that program an opportunity to work with you. It also gives you the opportunity to get a letter of recommendation from well-known people in that particular field.

Residency interviews take place in late fall and early winter of your fourth year. The main residency match occurs in March. For more information on specialties and the match see chapters 14 and 16.

USMLE Step 2 Clinical Knowledge (CK) exam and **Clinical Skills (CS) exam** are taken after you pass Step 1 and before you start your first year of residency. Most students take the exams sometime during their fourth year of medical school. Those who want to get it out of the way and those who want their score to appear on their residency application will take Step 2CK early in their fourth year. A step 2CK score was reported for 79% of residency applicants, with 73.2% of U.S. allopathic seniors reporting a Step 2CK score on their residency application (28).

Step 2CK is a nine-hour, computerized exam consisting of 352 questions. There are eight sections, each containing 44 questions. Examinees are given 60 minutes for each section and 60 minutes of total break time, rationed at the examinees' discretion throughout the day. If an examinee finishes a section early, the extra time is added to their break time. The exam is administered at Prometric™ testing centers throughout the world (87). The exam covers the pathophysiology, diagnosis and treatment of diseases and disorders that affect all organ systems. It also covers normal growth, development and aging. Nearly all topics should be covered during third year medical school clerkships. It currently costs $505 to take the exam (85). Once you pass the exam, you cannot take it again in an effort to achieve a higher score.

Step 2CK examinees are given a three digit score and a two digit score. The two-digit score is calculated from the three-digit score such that a passing score, 184, is equal to 75 (86). Most residency programs use the three-digit score, as it is more specific. The NBME no longer releases the percentile for each score. In "Charting Outcomes in the Match," the National Residency Matching Program (NRMP) stated the mean USMLE Step 2CK score of U.S. senior applicants and independent applicants, as well as the standard deviation of these scores (28). I calculated the "overall" mean step 2CK score and standard deviation from the number of each type of applicant, and the respective mean score and standard deviation.[14] Given the overall mean step 2CK score and standard deviation, and assuming the scores distribute themselves into a normal "Gaussian" distribution, I was able to calculate the "assumed" percentile of each score. These are not the actual percentiles; however, they can give you an idea as to what a "competitive" Step 2CK score is.

---

[14]   Among U.S. Seniors, the mean USMLE Step 2CK score was 229.7 and the standard deviation was 21.8. Among independent applicants, the mean USMLE Step 2CK score was 213.4 and the standard deviation was 21.3.
[(229.7 x 14958) + (213.4 x 13759)] / (14958 + 13759) = 221.9
[(21.8 x 14958) + (21.3 x 13759)] / (14958 + 13759) = 21.6

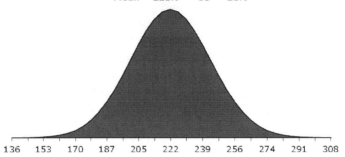

USMLE Step 2CK scores assuming a normal (Gaussian) distribution
Mean = 221.9   SD = 21.6

136   153   170   187   205   222   239   256   274   291   308

Table 12.2.   *USMLE Step 2 Score Percentiles assuming a normal (Gaussian) distribution*
SD = 21.6

Score	Percentile	Score	Percentile	Score	Percentile	Score	Percentile
<172	1	208	26	222	51	237	76
178	2	209	27	223	52	238	77
181	3	209	28	224	53	239	78
184	4	210	29	224	54	239	79
186	5	211	30	225	55	240	80
188	6	211	31	225	56	241	81
190	7	212	32	226	57	242	82
192	8	212	33	226	58	242	83
193	9	213	34	227	59	243	84
194	10	214	35	227	60	244	85
195	11	214	36	228	61	245	86
197	12	215	37	228	62	246	87
198	13	215	38	229	63	247	88
199	14	216	39	230	64	248	89
200	15	216	40	230	65	250	90
200	16	217	41	231	66	251	91
201	17	218	42	231	67	252	92
202	18	218	43	232	68	254	93
203	19	219	44	233	69	255	94
204	20	219	45	233	70	257	95
205	21	220	46	234	71	260	96
205	22	220	47	234	72	263	97
206	23	221	48	235	73	266	98
207	24	221	49	236	74	>272	99

Score	Percentile	Score	Percentile	Score	Percentile	Score	Percentile
207	25	222	50	236	75		

Step 2CS is an eight-hour exam consisting of 12 simulated patient encounters. The simulated patients are trained actors. Each encounter lasts a total of 25 minutes. Up to 15 minutes may be spent in the examining room with the patient. The remaining time is spent outside of the exam room typing a note that describes your findings and your plan. After you leave the patient's room you cannot go back in. The exam is administered at only five testing centers in the United States.[15] It currently costs $1,075 to take the exam, in addition to any travel expenses (85). Examinees are evaluated by the simulated patients and licensed physicians who read the examinee's notes. Their evaluation is based on data gathering, documentation, communication, interpersonal skills and spoken English proficiency. It is a pass/fail exam (87).

Alpha Omega Alpha (AOA) is a national medical honor society. Most allopathic medical schools have an AOA chapter. Criteria for being elected into AOA vary among chapters; however, only one-sixth of the class can be offered membership (88). Some chapters simply offer the top 15% of the class membership. Some chapters consider class rank in addition to other factors when selecting students for membership. Regardless of the criteria used, only students from the top quartile of the class are eligible for membership (88). Most chapters offer membership to students in the fall of their fourth year so it can be included in their residency application. Some chapters offer membership to a few students during their third year of medical school, an honor known as "Junior AOA." Being a member of AOA tells residency programs that you are in the top of your class and it will help you to land the residency position of your choice. Overall, 14.7% of U.S. Seniors reported being members of AOA on their ERAS application. Among the U.S. Seniors who successfully matched into the specialty of their choice, 15.3 were members of AOA (28).

Most medical students participate in some type of research project during medical school. 64.8% of graduating medical students reported participating in a research project with a faculty member and 38% reported authorship of a research paper submitted for publication (5). Research experience will make you a more competitive residency applicant, so long as you don't let doing research adversely affect your class rank and USMLE scores. As you can imagine, you won't have much time to waste during medical school. Spending time working on research projects takes time away from studying, sleeping and other activities. That being said, you need to be very careful in choosing a project and mentor. You want to find a project that interests you and one that you can complete and publish in a short amount of time. You also want to work with faculty members who can write letters of recommendation for residency.

---

[15]   Atlanta, Philadelphia, Chicago, Houston, Los Angeles

Volunteering during medical school is great. Some people find that volunteering during medical school provides some solidarity and motivation because it reminds them of why they went to medical school to begin with. Others allow it to become a distraction and an excuse to study less. You went to medical school to learn to help people as a physician. To be a competent physician you need to study and master the material presented to you by your medical school. Don't justify doing poorly in medical school because you spent too much time volunteering as an STD educator. Stay focused: you need to be a competent physician, not an experienced STD educator. STDs will still be infecting people when you are done with medical school; however, by then you will be able to educate people *and* prescribe them medications to cure them of their infection.

USMLE Step 3 is not taken during medical school; it is typically taken near the end of your first year of residency. It is a 16-hour computer-based exam consisting of 480 questions split up into two eight-hour days. The exam contains multiple-choice questions and computer-based case simulations. The computer-based case simulations test the examinees decision-making skills at each step in the care of the simulated patient. Step 3 is scored similarly to Step 1 and Step 2CK with a three-digit and two-digit score. A passing score on the USMLE Step 3 is 187 (86).

13   25 Specialties and 96 Subspecialties

Do not let anyone tell you that you don't have the "right" personality to be a physician. Medicine needs and accepts all personalities. Introverts, extroverts, narcissists, obsessive-compulsives and many others find a place in medicine. Of course, medical school admission committees do their best to keep the greedy, the immoral, the unethical, the cruel and the insensitive out of medical school.

Medical licensure is the minimum requirement a physician needs to diagnose and treat patients in most states. Board certification demonstrates competence and expertise in a particular specialty or subspecialty (89). Physicians become eligible for board certification in a specialty after successfully completing an ACGME accredited residency program in that specialty. Physicians become board certified after completing a specialty-specific written board examination after residency. Some specialties also have an oral board examination in which candidates are grilled by leaders in the field to assess their competency and decision-making. To maintain board certification, physicians must re-certify every six to ten years depending on the specialty.

You may hear people talk about how the United States needs more primary care physicians, not more specialists. What they mean is that the United States needs more people to go into primary care specialties such as Family Medicine, Internal Medicine and Pediatrics. A board-certified Family Physician is board certified in the specialty of Family Medicine.

The American Board of Medical Specialties' (AMBS) 24 specialty boards certify physicians in more than 145 allopathic specialties and subspecialties (89).

After successfully completing an ACGME accredited residency training program, physicians become eligible for board certification in that specialty. After completing a fellowship, physicians become eligible for board certification in that subspecialty.

Table 13.1 is comprehensive but not all-inclusive. Specialties are in bold, and their respective subspecialties are in regular text below them. The first year of residency, known as internship, is included in the duration of training. The duration of training is the minimum number of years in which the training can be completed. For example, most general surgery residency programs are 5 years long. Some general surgery programs are 7 years long because they require 2 years of research at some point in residency. 5 years is the minimum amount of training required to be eligible for board certification in general surgery, so 5 years is used in the table below.

Some specialties, particularly surgical subspecialties, have been changed from fellowships after general surgery to "integrated" residency programs. Many plastic surgery fellowship programs have converted to 6-year integrated plastic surgery residency programs. There are now integrated vascular surgery and thoracic surgery residency programs as well. This means that there are two paths to becoming a plastic surgeon, vascular surgeon or thoracic surgeon; you can take the more direct "integrated" residency-training route or the traditional fellowship route after completing a general surgery residency.

Are fellowships necessary? It depends. General surgeons are trained in vascular surgery, trauma surgery, pediatric surgery and thoracic surgery. At the time they complete their residency they are capable of performing some vascular surgery procedures, some thoracic surgery procedures, and so on. Doing a fellowship will give them a significant amount of additional training in that particular area, which will allow them to do more complex procedures and earn board certification in that subspecialty. In order to get hospital privileges and malpractice insurance to perform vascular surgery, you probably need to be a fellowship trained vascular surgeon in most circumstances. In a smaller, secluded rural hospital you may be able to get hospital privileges and malpractice insurance to perform some vascular surgery procedures as a general surgeon without fellowship training in vascular surgery.

An explanation of each allopathic specialty and subspecialty would be as boring as Appendix 1 and far less useful. Table 13.1 is useful if you are trying to decide whether or not to become a physician, because eventually you will have to choose one of the specialties and possibly a subspecialty. However, reading through a description of each specialty and subspecialty would be a little premature. Table 13.1 is useful if you are a medical student because it lays out all the options to help get you started on your quest to figure out what you should do for the rest of your life. If you want to learn more about certain specialties and subspecialties, do some research online and try to spend some time with a physician in that field.

Table 13.1. *Allopathic Specialties and Subspecialties*

Specialty	Residency training *after* medical school (years)	Average hours worked per week *after* residency (90)	Median Gross Income (30, 35)	Median Net Income[16] (91)	Adjusted Net Hourly Wage[17] ($)
Anesthesiology	4	61	366,640	230,987	53
Critical Care Medicine	5		*268,250*	*176,820*	
Hospice & Palliative Medicine	5				
Pain Medicine	5				
Dermatology	4	45.5	350,627	222,165	62
Dermatopathology	5				
Pediatric Dermatology	5				
Mohs Micrographic Surgery	5				
Emergency Medicine	3	46	267,293	176,293	50
Hospice & Palliative Medicine	4				
Medical Toxicology	5				
Pediatric Emergency Medicine	6				
Sports Medicine	4		*214,249*	*146,228*	
Undersea & Hyperbaric Medicine	4				
Family Medicine	3	52.5	197,655	136,264	34
Adolescent Medicine	6		*202,832*	*139,373*	
Geriatric Medicine	4		*144,531*	*211,425*	
Hospice & Palliative Medicine	4				
Sleep Medicine	4				
Sports Medicine	4		*214,249*	*146,228*	
Internal Medicine	3	57	205,441	140,939	34
Allergy & Immunology	5		*241,138*	*161,896*	
Cardiology	6		*398,034*	*248,219*	
Interventional Cardiology	7				
Clinical Cardiac Electrophysiology	8				
Heart Failure & Transplant Cardiology	7				
Pulmonary Disease & Critical Care Medicine	6		*278,000*	*182,186*	
Sleep Medicine	4				
Endocrinology	5		*212,281*	*145,046*	
Adolescent Medicine	6		*202,832*	*139,373*	
Gastroenterology	6		*389,385*	*243,498*	

[16] Calculated based on 2010 income tax rates for someone living in California, married, with two children and opting out of the California state disability insurance. Calculation performed at *www.paycheckcity.com*. Federal Income Tax varies with gross income (see Tables 6.1 and 6.2). California 2010 personal income tax rate of 6.6%.

[17] Assuming you graduate from medical school at 23 years old and work the average number of hours listed for 48 weeks each year until you are 65 years old. Assuming you work 80 hours per week, 50 weeks per year in residency and receive a net annual salary of $40,000. Assuming you attended average priced institutions, took out loans to pay all costs, forbore your loans in residency and paid them off over 20 years at 7% APR.

Specialty	Residency training *after* medical school (years)	Average hours worked per week *after* residency (90)	Median Gross Income (30, 35)	Median Net Income[16] (91)	Adjusted Net Hourly Wage[17] ($)
Geriatric Medicine	*4*		*211,425*	*144,531*	
Hematology & Oncology	*6*		*315,133*	*202,627*	
Hospice & Palliative Medicine	*4*				
Infectious Disease	*5*		*222,094*	*150,938*	
Nephrology	*5*		*246,049*	*164,599*	
Rheumatology	*5*		*219,411*	*149,327*	
Transplant Hepatology	*4*				
Sports Medicine	*4*		*214,249*	*146,228*	
Clinical Genetics (92)	4				
Medical Biochemical Genetics	*5*				
Molecular Genetic Pathology	*5*				
Neurosurgery	7		548,186	327,867	
Pediatric Neurosurgery	*8*				
Spine Surgery	*8*		*641,728*	*377,487*	
Neuroendovascular Surgery	*9*				
Child Neurology	5		209,955	143,649	
Neurology	4	55.5	236,500	159,343	38
Clinical Neurophysiology	*5*				
Hospice & Palliative Medicine	*5*[18]				
Neuromuscular Medicine	*5*[19]				
Pain Medicine	*5*				
Sleep Medicine	*5*[20]				
Vascular Neurology	*5*				
Neuro-ophthalmology	*5*				
Nuclear Medicine[21] (93)	5		414,500	256,953	
Obstetrics & Gynecology	4	61	294,190	191,099	43
Critical Care Medicine	*5*		*268,250*	*176,820*	
Gynecologic Oncology	*7*		*406,000*	*252,444*	
Hospice & Palliative Medicine	*5*				
Maternal & Fetal Medicine	*7*				
Reproductive Endocrinology & Infertility	*7*		*317,943*	*204,173*	
Female Pelvic Medicine & Reconstructive Surgery	*7*				
Ophthalmology	4	47	325,384	208,270	57
Oculoplastic Surgery	*6*				

---

18   After 2012
19   After 2012
20   After 2011
21   Certification in Nuclear Medicine can be earned by completing 2 years of training after become eligible for board certification in another specialty such as internal medicine, family medicine, pediatrics, etc. Physicians who will be board certified in Radiology need only complete 1 year of nuclear medicine training.

Specialty	Residency training *after* medical school (years)	Average hours worked per week *after* residency (90)	Median Gross Income (30, 35)	Median Net Income[16] (91)	Adjusted Net Hourly Wage[17] ($)
Vitreoretinal Surgery	6				
Neuro-ophthalmology	5				
Plastic & Reconstructive Surgery	7				
Oral Surgery	6[22]		400,000	249,262	
Orthopedic Surgery	5	58	476,083	289,620	67
Orthopedic Sports Medicine	6				
Surgery of the Hand	6		*465,006*	*283,744*	
Orthopedic Foot & Ankle Surgery	6				
Spine Surgery			*641,728*	*377,487*	
Pediatric Orthopedic Surgery	6		*424,367*	*262,187*	
Otolaryngology (ENT)	5	53.5	365,171	230,170	55
Neurotology	7				
Pediatric Otolaryngology	6				
Plastic Surgery Within the Head & Neck	6				
Sleep Medicine	6				
Plastic & Reconstructive Surgery	8				
Pathology – Anatomic & Clinical	4	45.5	344,195	218,624	61
Blood Banking & Transfusion Medicine	5				
Cytopathology	5				
Dermatopathology	5				
Neuropathology	6				
Clinical Chemistry	6				
Forensic Pathology	5				
Hematopathology	5				
Clinical Microbiology	5				
Molecular Pathology	5				
Pediatric Pathology	5				
Surgical Pathology	5				
Pediatrics	3	54	202,832	139,373	35
Adolescent Medicine	6		*202,832*	*139,373*	
Child Abuse Pediatrics	6				
Developmental - Behavioral Pediatrics	6				
Hospice & Palliative Medicine	4				
Medical Toxicology	5				
Neonatal-Perinatal Medicine	6		*265,000*	*175,031*	
Allergy & Immunology	5		*241,138*	*161,896*	

---

[22] Oral Surgery: Dental School (4) + Medical School (2) + Residency (4) = 10.   10 – 4 (traditional medical school) = 6. The equivalent of 6 years of additional, post-medical school training.

Specialty	Residency training *after* medical school (years)	Average hours worked per week *after* residency (90)	Median Gross Income (30, 35)	Median Net Income[16] (91)	Adjusted Net Hourly Wage[17] ($)
Pediatric Cardiology	6		*244,944*	*163,991*	
Pediatric Critical Care Medicine	6		*265,913*	*175,533*	
Pediatric Emergency Medicine	6				
Pediatric Endocrinology	6		*185,901*	*129,206*	
Pediatric Gastroenterology	6		*236,700*	*159,453*	
Pediatric Hematology & Oncology	6		*205,999*	*141,274*	
Pediatric Infectious Diseases	6		*199,165*	*137,170*	
Pediatric Nephrology	6		*217,767*	*148,340*	
Pediatric Pulmonology	6		*176,974*	*123,846*	
Pediatric Rheumatology	6				
Pediatric Transplant Hepatology	7				
Sleep Medicine	4				
Sports Medicine	4		*214,249*	*146,228*	
Physical Medicine & Rehabilitation	4		236,500	159,343	
Hospice & Palliative Medicine	5				
Neuromuscular Medicine	5[23]				
Pain Medicine	5				
Pediatric Rehabilitation Medicine	6				
Spinal Cord Injury Medicine	5				
Sports Medicine	5		*214,249*	*146,228*	
Plastic & Reconstructive Surgery	6		388,929	243,248	
Surgery of the Hand	7		*465,006*	*283,744*	
Microsurgery	7				
Craniofacial Surgery	7				
Preventative Medicine(94)	3				
Medical Toxicology(95)	5				
Undersea & Hyperbaric Medicine (95)	4				
Psychiatry	4	48	208,462	142,753	37
Child & Adolescent Psychiatry	5		*214,304*	*146,260*	
Addiction Psychiatry	5				
Forensic Psychiatry	5				
Geriatric Psychiatry	5				
Hospice & Palliative Medicine	5[24]				
Pain Medicine	5				
Psychosomatic Medicine	5				
Sleep Medicine	5[25]				

[23] After 2013
[24] After 2012
[25] After 2011

Specialty	Residency training *after* medical school (years)	Average hours worked per week *after* residency (90)	Median Gross Income (30, 35)	Median Net Income[16] (91)	Adjusted Net Hourly Wage[17] ($)
Radiation Oncology	4		413,518	256,432	
Diagnostic Radiology	5	58	438,115	269,480	62
Hospice & Palliative Medicine	6				
Neuroradiology	6				
Nuclear Medicine	6		*414,500*	*256,953*	
Pediatric Radiology	6				
Vascular & Interventional Radiology	6		*478,000*	*290,636*	
General Surgery	5	60	340,000	216,314	48
Colon & Rectal Surgery	6		*366,895*	*231,119*	
Vascular Surgery	7		*403,041*	*250,875*	
Thoracic Surgery	7		*507,143*	*306,095*	
Plastic & Reconstructive Surgery	8		*388,929*	*243,248*	
Surgery of the Hand	6		*465,006*	*283,744*	
Surgical Critical Care	6		*268,250*	*176,820*	
Surgical Critical Care & Trauma Surgery	7		*465,773*	*284,151*	
Pediatric Surgery	7		*400,591*	*249,576*	
Transplant Surgery	7		*433,333*	*266,943*	
Breast Surgery	6				
Surgical Oncology	7				
Minimally Invasive Surgery	6				
Thoracic Surgery	6		507,143	306,095	
Urology	5	60.5	389,198	243,396	54
Pediatric Urology	7				
Female Pelvic Medicine & Reconstructive Surgery	8				
Plastic & Reconstructive Surgery	8				
Vascular Surgery	5		403,041	250,875	

While the American Board of Medical Specialties (ABMS) certifies physicians in allopathic specialties and subspecialties, the American Osteopathic Association's Bureau of Osteopathic Specialists oversees 18 AOA osteopathic specialty-certifying boards. Osteopathic medical school graduates may train in AOA approved osteopathic residency programs or ACGME approved allopathic residency programs. Depending on which type of residency they complete, they may become board certified through the AMBS or the AOA. There are "Dual Programs," which are residency programs approved by both the AOA and the ACGME. Osteopathic physicians who graduate from these dual programs are eligible for board certification by the AMBS, AOA or both (96).

In 2009 there were 2,435 accredited osteopathic residency-training positions for the 3,724 osteopathic medical school seniors. However, only 1,794 osteopathic seniors applied for osteopathic residency training positions and 1,433 of these applicants successfully matched into an osteopathic residency training position (97). It is assumed that the other 1,930 osteopathic medical school seniors who didn't enter the osteopathic residency match applied only for allopathic residency positions. On average, about 60% of osteopathic medical school graduates go on to train in allopathic (ACGME) residency programs and 40% go on to train in osteopathic (AOA) residency programs (98, 99). See chapter 16 for information on the Osteopathic Residency Match. See table 16.2 for more information about osteopathic applicants applying for allopathic residencies.

21 Osteopathic Specialties and 26 Osteopathic Subspecialties (98, 99):

Anesthesiology
   Pain Management
Dermatology
   Mohs Micrographic Surgery
Diagnostic Radiology
   Vascular Interventional Radiology
Emergency Medicine
Family Practice
   Geriatrics
   Sports Medicine
Internal Medicine & Pediatrics
Internal Medicine
   Geriatrics
   Sports Medicine
   Cardiology
      Electrophysiology
      Interventional
   Critical Care Medicine
   Endocrinology
   Gastroenterology
   Hematology & Oncology
   Infectious Diseases
   Nephrology
   Oncology
   Pulmonary Medicine
   Pulmonary and Critical Care Medicine
   Rheumatology

Neurology
Neuromusculoskeletal Medicine
Obstetrics & Gynecology
   Gynecologic Oncology
   Maternal & Fetal Medicine
   Reproductive Endocrinology
Ophthalmology
Orthopedic Surgery
   Hand Surgery
   Orthopedic Spine Surgery
Otolaryngology & Facial Plastic Surgery
Pediatrics
   Pediatric Allergy & Immunology
Physical Medicine & Rehabilitation
Preventative Medicine & Public Health
Proctology
Psychiatry
   Child Psychiatry
General Surgery
   Cardiothoracic Surgery
   Vascular Surgery
   Plastic & Reconstructive Surgery
Neurological Surgery
Urological Surgery

14   Choosing a Specialty

Deciding what you will do after medical school and for the rest of your life is an important decision. At 27 years old, your life expectancy is 81 years old (3). If you sleep an average of 7 hours each night, you have 335,070 waking hours left to live. You will spend about 6% of your remaining waking life training in whichever specialty you choose, and 27% of your remaining waking life practicing that specialty. Therefore, what you do for about ONE THIRD of your remaining waking life will be determined by the specialty you choose. To make things more difficult, this decision needs to be made before the end of your third year of medical school, prior to requesting your fourth year schedule. This doesn't give you much time after you start your clinical rotations to figure it out, so you should start pondering and exploring early.

When trying to figure out what to go into, you need to first think about what excites you. What do you want to do for one-third of your remaining waking life? What do you want to go home and read about at night? What is your passion?

You may want more from your life than simply your career, so think about how you will fit your family in; or, more appropriately, how the specialty you choose will fit into the family life you envision. Unfortunately, more demanding specialties such as neurosurgery or transplant surgery are more difficult to fit into the rest of your life than less demanding specialties like dermatology or radiology. However, your family and friends would probably prefer to see you less but have you happy than see you more but have you miserable. Don't go into something you don't particularly like because you think it will be less demanding.

You also need to consider your age and the length of training. As you saw in chapter 4, age and infertility can sneak up on you. What would you resent more: not being able to have children of your own or not being able to be a cardiologist?

Should you let money influence your decision? The morally correct answer is: no, you should not! In reality, however, most medical students do let money influence their decision, as 75% admitted that income expectations influenced their decision (5). A large minority of students, 45%, reported that their student debt influenced their decision (5).

Yes, you can change specialties, but, if you look at the data in table 16.2, you will see that it is generally easier to match into residency programs as a medical school senior than as a medical school graduate. Moreover, the longer you put off figuring out what you want to do, the longer the process takes and the more debt you will have. Of course, things cannot always be planned perfectly, no matter how hard you try. If you thought you wanted to be a general surgeon, but didn't realize that you would actually rather be an anesthesiologist until you are a general surgery resident – that is ok. You can change, but it is a more difficult process than matching into anesthesiology as a senior medical student.

If you read any books, articles or handouts about choosing a medical specialty, you will probably see the specialty satisfaction list in table 14.1.

Table 14.1. *Overall Career Satisfaction (51)*

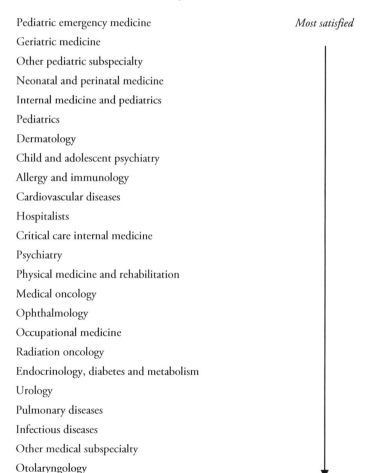

Pediatric emergency medicine   *Most satisfied*
Geriatric medicine
Other pediatric subspecialty
Neonatal and perinatal medicine
Internal medicine and pediatrics
Pediatrics
Dermatology
Child and adolescent psychiatry
Allergy and immunology
Cardiovascular diseases
Hospitalists
Critical care internal medicine
Psychiatry
Physical medicine and rehabilitation
Medical oncology
Ophthalmology
Occupational medicine
Radiation oncology
Endocrinology, diabetes and metabolism
Urology
Pulmonary diseases
Infectious diseases
Other medical subspecialty
Otolaryngology

General practice

Family practice

Gastroenterology

Internal medicine

Other surgical subspecialty

General surgery

Neurology

Plastic surgery

Rheumatology

Orthopedic surgery

Emergency medicine

Thoracic surgery

Hematology and oncology

Vascular surgery

Obstetrics and gynecology

Nephrology

Pulmonary critical care medicine

Neurological surgery   *Least satisfied*

I present this list to explain why this information is *not* very helpful. It does not tell you what specialty is most satisfying, it tells you which types of physicians are most satisfied. It illustrates that a geriatrician is more likely to report being satisfied than a neurosurgeon. It is not becoming a geriatrician that necessarily makes people satisfied, but rather that the type of people who go into geriatrics are more likely to report being satisfied than the type of people who go into neurosurgery. It has more to do with the type of personality that a specialty attracts than the specialty itself causing satisfaction. If you were to take a hundred neurosurgeons and force them to become geriatricians, I doubt you would make them more satisfied. This is not to say that geriatricians are better people than neurosurgeons. Neither the specialty nor the type of personality it attracts is "better" than the other. This illustrates the point that medicine needs and accepts all personalities. If my brain is bleeding and I am about to die, I want a neurosurgeon and the type of people neurosurgery attracts to be cutting my head open. When I am elderly, frail and full of chronic medical problems; I want a patient, kind geriatrician to listen to me talk about my ailments and my grandchildren. All personalities have a place; you just need to find yours. You should pick a specialty that is most likely to make YOU satisfied, which is not necessarily the specialty that has the most satisfied people.

The Association of American Medical Colleges (AAMC) developed a career planning program known as "Careers in Medicine" (CiM). Unfortunately, it does not hold "your answer," but it may help you in your decision making process. 40% of the 2009 graduating allopathic medical school class reported that the "Careers in Medicine" website had a moderate or strong influence on their specialty choice (5) (*http://www.aamc.org/students/cim/start.htm*).

If you are frustrated and confused because you can't figure out what to do, you are not alone. Most medical students have some difficulty figuring out what to specialize in. About 50% of allopathic medical school graduates reported being unsatisfied with the career planning services at their medical school (5).

Heed the advice of others, especially your spouse or partner, but do not let yourself be swayed or bullied into a specialty by anyone. It is your life and your career, and you will be the one who has to live with your decision.

15 Residency Application

Applications to most residency and fellowship programs are submitted via the Electronic Residency Application Service (ERAS). For a list of participating specialties and their respective programs go to https://services.aamc.org/eras/erasstats/par/index.cfm.

Application deadlines vary by program. In general, if a program has many training positions to fill, they will need to interview and rank many applicants. In order to fit in a large number of interviews, they must start early, and consequently their application deadline will be earlier than a program that has only a few positions to fill.

The application process is separate from the matching process. ERAS© compiles, manages and distributes your application to residency programs. Applicants are matched into residency positions through the military match, urology match, osteopathic match, San Francisco match and the "main" NRMP© match. ERAS© registration and fees are separate from matching service registration and fees. In the fall of your fourth year you need to register with both ERAS© and the matching service you will be using.

In order to match into a residency, you need to be ranked highly enough by a residency program. In order to be ranked highly enough by a residency program, you have to go through an interview there and leave a good impression. In order to be offered an interview, you have to have a good application. The content of your application will reflect what you have done over many years, so it is worthwhile to know what the components of the residency application are. ERAS© Application Components:

Profile

- Name
- Preferred name
- Medical School
- Birth date
- E-mail address
- Postal address
- Phone number
- Citizenship

- Visa Type
- USMLE ID number
- NBOME ID number (osteopathic applicants)
- American Osteopathic Association member number (osteopathic applicants)
- American Urological Association ID number (Urology applicants)
- ECFMG Certification Status
- Planning to participate in the National Residency Matching Program?
  - Select: yes/no
- Applying as a couple?
  - Select: Yes/no.
  - If yes: partner's name and specialties they are applying to
- Alpha Omega Alpha Medical Honor Society Status
  - Select: Member/Elections held during senior year/No AOA chapter at my school/Not a member
- Sigma Sigma Phi Status (osteopathic applicants)
  - Select: Member/Elections held during senior year/No SSP chapter at my school/Not a member
- ECFMG certification status

Common Application Form (CAF) – cannot be changed after it is certified

- Service obligations (military, National Health Service Corps, etc.)
- Undergraduate and graduate institutions attended before medical school
  - Major
  - Dates Attended
  - Degrees earned or expected
- Medical Schools Attended
  - Dates Attended
  - Degrees earned or expected
- Prior Graduate Medical Education or Training
- Experiences
  - Select: Work / Research / Volunteer
  - Organization
  - Location
  - Position
  - Supervisor
  - Average hours per week
  - Dates
  - Reason for leaving
- Publications

- o Select: Published Peer Reviewed Journal Article / Submitted Peer Reviewed Journal Article / Peer Reviewed Book Chapter / Scientific Monograph / Other Articles / Poster Presentation / Oral Presentation / Peer Reviewed Online Publication / Non Peer Reviewed Online Publication
  - o Fill in relevant data depending on type of publication
- Medical Licensure Information
- Language Fluency other than English
  - o If you fill in a language, you should be able to interview in that language.
- Hobbies and Interests (510 characters)
- Medical School Awards (510 characters)
- Other Awards / Accomplishments (510 characters)
- Membership in Honorary/Professional Societies (255 characters)

Documents

- Medical School Transcript
- USMLE Transcript or Score Report
  - o Your USMLE transcript contains all exams taken, available scores, failed attempts, special test accommodations and any actions taken against you by medical licensing authorities. Your personal graphical performance profiles are not included.
  - o Decide if you want ERAS to automatically transmit an updated USMLE score report when new USMLE exam results become available. If you check "no," you can always go back and check "yes," if, after viewing your new scores, you decide you would like them released to programs.
  - o Each time that you assign your USMLE transcript to a program, your most recent transcript will be uploaded.
- Medical Student Performance Evaluation (MSPE)
  - o Formerly known as the "Dean's Letter." Your MSPE is written and submitted by your medical school along with your transcript. It contains a fair and objective evaluation of your overall performance in medical school. The MSPE typically contains attending physician comments from your clerkship evaluations. It will also mention distinguishing characteristics, hardships, leaves of absence, repeated coursework, etc.
- COMLEX Transcript (osteopathic students).
- ECFMG Status Report (International Medical Graduates).
  - o Postgraduate Training Authorization Letter (PTAL) or "California Letter" (International Medical Graduates).
- 5th Pathway Certificate (International Medical Graduates)

- Photo
  - Only one photo. Can only submit once.
  - Less than 3 x 4 inches.
  - When the faculty of a residency program meet to generate their applicant rank list, they will rely on this photograph to couple your application with how you came across during the interview. "Oh, I remember eating dinner with this guy/gal…" That being said, submit a recent photograph that looks like you and remember: a picture is worth a thousand words.
- Personal Statements
  - Limited to 28,000 characters. However, many faculty frown on personal statements longer than one page, or 3,500 characters.
  - You may attach only one personal statement to each program.
  - In your personal statement you need to explain your life's mission. What are you going to do with your training? How will you contribute to the field?
- Letters of Recommendation
  - Always give potential letter writers the option to decline your request. "Dr. Smith, would you be comfortable writing a strong letter of recommendation on my behalf?"
  - Print coversheets for your letter writers.
  - List and reserve a "slot" in ERAS for the individuals that will be submitting Letters of recommendations on your behalf.
  - IMGs must designate a "slot" in ERAS for their California Letter.
  - Assign up to 4 Letters of recommendations to each residency program.
  - Waive your right to read it. If you don't, many residency programs will assume you are trying to hide something.

Programs to which you are applying

- Attach one personal statement to each program.
- Attach up to 4 letters of recommendation to each program.
- Programs cannot see which other programs you applied to.

16 The Residency Match

The residency application process starts with filling out your application online via the Electronic Residency Application Service© (ERAS). This application is described in chapter 15. Through ERAS, you select which residency programs you want to apply to. Your application is then sent electronically to the programs you select. Residency programs that are interested in you offer you an interview and you then interview at as many programs as you can. In February of your senior year, after interview season, you will submit a program "rank list" to the National Residency Matching Program© (NRMP) or whichever matching service you are using. Residency programs also submit their applicant "rank lists" and a matching process takes place. So, you apply to residency through ERAS and are matched into a program through the NRMP or other matching program.

A few specialties do not use the NRMP. Ophthalmology and Pediatric Neurology use the San Francisco Matching Program©. The American Urological Association© (AUA) conducts the Urology match. Military and osteopathic residency programs have their own matching process.

In 2009 the NRMP enrolled 4,299 programs which offered 25,185 training positions (72). 95.4% of these positions were filled (73). A total of 36,972 applicants participated in the match (73). 15,638 were U.S. allopathic medical school seniors (28), 1,222 had previously graduated from U.S. allopathic medical schools (28), 2,013 were seniors or graduates of osteopathic medical schools (28), 3,390 were U.S. citizens who graduated from International Medical Schools (28), and 7,484 were non-U.S. citizen graduates of International Medical Schools (28).

In 2009, 71.4% of applicants successfully matched into a residency training position (73). U.S. allopathic medical school seniors had the highest match rate, at 93.1%, with about half of them matching into their first choice (73). Osteopathic medical school seniors and graduates had the next highest match rate of 69.9% (73). U.S. Citizens who have or will graduate from foreign medical schools had a 47.8% match rate (73). Former graduates of U.S. allopathic medical schools had a 44.6% match rate (73). Non-U.S. citizen students and graduates of foreign medical schools had a 41.6% match rate (73).

If you apply to a specialty that utilizes the NRMP, you will submit your residency program "rank list" at the end of February. Programs will also submit their applicant "rank list" at that time. After rank lists from both parties have been submitted, the match algorithm starts running. You will then anxiously wait until the middle of March to learn your fate.

Before I explain the match algorithm, I want to explain the different types of residency training positions, which includes categorical positions, advanced positions and preliminary positions. Categorical positions are those that provide applicants with all the years of graduate medical education they need in order to become eligible for board certification in that specialty. Advanced positions are those that provide applicants with all the graduate medical education they need in order to become eligible for board certification in that specialty, except for the PGY-1 year, or intern year. For example, many radiology programs expect applicants to obtain a PGY-1 training position separately. So, if in March of 2011 a medical school senior matches into an advanced radiology training position, they are matching into a position that starts in July of 2012 with the expectation that they will have completed an internship by that time. Those who apply for advanced residency positions must also apply for preliminary positions. Preliminary positions provide one year, sometimes two years, of graduate medical education as a pre-requisite to an advanced residency position. Preliminary positions do not offer the training necessary to become eligible for board certification in any specialty. Preliminary years are typically designated as "internal medicine," "surgery," or "transitional." Completing a preliminary "internal medicine" year is similar to completing the first year of a categorical internal medicine residency. Completing a preliminary "surgery" year is similar to completing the first year of a categorical surgery residency. Transitional preliminary years tend to offer more variety and often have their interns rotate on medical services, surgical services and pediatric services.

To explain the match algorithm, I'll use a hypothetical applicant named John who is trying to match into a Pediatrics residency. His first choice is Mercury, his second is Venus, his third is Earth, and so on. The match algorithm starts with trying to place John into his first choice, Mercury. However, Mercury didn't even rank John, so the algorithm moves on to Venus. Venus ranked John so he is "tentatively" offered a position, which John will never know about. The algorithm then continues with other applicants. As the algorithm continues, Venus ends up filling its training positions with applicants who are higher on Venus's rank list than John. John then gets bumped to Earth. Earth ranked John, and John is ranked higher on Earth's list than 3 of the applicants "tentatively" matched to Earth, so the least desirable of these 3 applicants gets bumped off Earth and move down their list, while John stays on earth. The match algorithm continues until every applicant's rank list has been run through the algorithm.

Ultimately, the algorithm creates the best theoretical combination among applicants and programs. If you rank a program that has 3 positions #1 and they rank you #1, #2 or #3 – you will match there. If you rank a program that has 3 positions #1 and they rank you #6, you have to hope that 3 of those 5 applicants who are ranked higher than you match elsewhere. They will match elsewhere if they ranked another program higher and if this other program ranked them high enough that they will match there. If applicants and programs make their rank lists from their first choice to their last choice, regardless of how good their "chances" are, the best theoretical combination for everyone will work itself out. If Mercury is your first choice but you know it is a long shot, you have nothing to lose by not ranking it your #1.

Many people find love within their medical school class. The NRMP respects this and developed a special "couples' match" algorithm for these applicants. Each party registers with the NRMP individually but indicates that they want to participate in the match as a couple. They then enter information to identify the applicant with whom they hope to match. Couples can make a list of up to 30 pairs that can include any combination of programs, specialties and the willingness to go unmatched if the other partner matches at a particular program. The couple will match into their most preferred pair. Supplemental individual rank order lists are prepared for preliminary positions. The coupling algorithm is only run for the primary list of the couple. If a couple wants to match into dermatology and radiology, both of which require completion of a preliminary year, they will "couple's match" for dermatology and radiology but will have to match individually for the preliminary year positions.

Couples are more likely to match successfully if they choose specialties with many training positions and apply to programs in large cities where they can maximize the number of workable program pairs.

A couple's rank order list might look like this:

Table 16.1. Example of the Couples' Match Rank Order List

Partner 1	Partner 2
New York City – Internal Medicine A	New York City – Pediatrics A
New York City – Internal Medicine A	New York City – Pediatrics B
New York City – Internal Medicine B	New York City – Pediatrics A
New York City – Internal Medicine B	New York City – Pediatrics B
Chicago – Internal Medicine C	Chicago – Pediatrics C
San Francisco – Internal Medicine D	Oakland – Pediatrics D
New York City – Internal Medicine A	No Match
No Match	New York City – Pediatrics A
... up to 30 pairs	*... up to 30 pairs*

In deciding to match as a couple, you must decide if the relationship is more important than your career. This is a very difficult decision that many couples face at the beginning of their fourth year. When you match as a couple you will keep falling down your rank list until you both match into one of your paired combinations. For example, if you were ranked to match by all three of your top programs but your partner was not ranked to match by any of the programs that were paired with your top 3 programs, you will not match into any of those programs. You will continue falling down your rank list until a program picks up both you and your partner, so he or she better be worth it.

However, matching with a partner who is a stronger applicant than you may help you out even though you will drag them down. Residency programs within a city or region have been known to bargain with each other. Let's take a hypothetical couple who we'll call Jack and Jill. Jill is a superstar applicant, while Jack is a fair applicant. Program A really wants Jill, but they know that in order to get Jill, they have to get Jack accepted into some program in the same city. Fortunately, Chairman of Program A has a friend who is the residency director at a program Jack applied to, so Chairman of Program A calls this residency director and kindly encourages them to consider taking Jack.

In 2009, 788 couples participated in the main residency match. For 706 couples, both parties matched. For 55 couples, one of them matched. For 27 couples, neither matched. This is an overall match rate of about 93%, the same as the match rate among all U.S. Allopathic Medical school seniors (73). As you can see, couples' matching has no intrinsic benefits; in fact, it has only statistical disadvantages. I think the reason the couples match rate is the same as the overall U.S. allopathic medical school senior match rate is because people who couples match are more strategic and conservative in playing the match game than solo applicants. Because applicants who are couples matching start at a statistical disadvantage, they apply to more programs, go on more interviews and ultimately are able to rank more programs such that, in the end, they are equally as successful as their single counterparts.

Unfortunately, if one or both parties of "the couple" are trying to match into urology, ophthalmology or pediatric neurology, they will be unable to couples match. In order to couples match the "couples' algorithm" has to be run and this is only possible if both parties are going into specialties that use the NRMP.

On the Monday of match week, in the middle of March, after the match algorithm as been run, you will be notified of whether or not you successfully matched. If you did, you must wait until Thursday to find out where. If you didn't match, then, with the help of your advisors, you need to figure out what you should do. One option is doing research and applying again next year. If you do this, then the question is: should you graduate and become a U.S. allopathic graduate or stay in medical school for another year to remain a "senior." Another option is to scramble into a vacant training position. On the Monday of match week, if you get the bad news that you didn't match, you will have the opportunity to re-submit applications through ERAS to 30 programs with vacancies. Then, from Tuesday 11:30am through Thursday 12pm, phone calls among scrambling applicants and programs take place. Only applicants who entered the NRMP and failed to match are eligible to scramble. Unmatched applicants can scramble into categorical, advanced and/or preliminary positions. After Thursday 12pm, program vacancies are then open to all applicants, regardless of whether or not they participated in the match. If you scramble into a preliminary position without an appointment in an advanced position, you will have to find a vacancy somewhere or re-enter the match next year with the intent of matching into a categorical or advanced position. If you then match into a categorical position, you may have to repeat your intern year. If you match into an advanced position, you will likely have to wait one more year before you can start, because advanced positions start about 15 months after the match. The costs of not matching are higher than the costs of applying to many programs and interviewing at many programs, so it is best to play the game conservatively even if you are a superstar.

In order to play the match game effectively, it is helpful to have an appreciation of how competitive a specialty is, based on the match rate for various types of applicants and the characteristics of those applicants who successfully match. Table 16.2 contains match rates by specialty and applicant type. The match rate data from the NRMP only distinguishes U.S. allopathic seniors from all others. These "others" are called independent applicants. The NRMP did, however, release the number of each type of independent applicant who matched into each specialty, but they did not release the number of applicants of each type of independent applicant, so match rates could not be calculated.

INFORMED CONSENT

Table 16.2. *2009 Allopathic Residency Match (28, 73, 100-102)*

Specialty	Training Positions	Total # Applicants	Match Rate U.S. Allopathic Seniors	Match Rate Independent Applicants	# Independent Applicants Matched			
					U.S. Allopathic Grads	D.O.	U.S. IMG	IMG
Thoracic Surgery[26]	3	19	23%	0%	0	0	0	0
Vascular Surgery[26]	19	66	47%	12%	0	0	0	4
Plastic Surgery[26]	101	191	53%	41%	7	1	1	3
Dermatology	388	567	70%	31%	39	1	1	7
Urology	264	373	77%		27%	5	18%	7
Orthopedic Surgery	641	923	79%	30%	33	5	3	12
Otolaryngology (ENT)	275	373	80%	21%	5	0	2	3
Neurosurgery	191	295	80%	24%	3	1	3	12
General Surgery	1,065	1,630	85%	30%	76	31	48	78
Diagnostic Radiology	1,095	1,477	86%	34%	39	39	21	37
Radiation Oncology	156	179	87%	33%	4	1	1	2
Child Neurology	181	148	89%	-	98%		86%	
Ophthalmology	459	654	92%		5%		3%	
Anesthesiology	1,374	1,729	92%	42%	34	101	52	50
Obstetrics & Gynecology	1,185	1,591	93%	44%	31	108	85	69
Emergency Medicine	1,515	1,817	93%	55%	58	171	78	21
Psychiatry	1,063	1,563	94%	42%	31	102	93	162
Pathology	522	708	94%	44%	27	34	29	80
Internal Medicine/Pediatrics	354	393	94%	57%	8	27	28	35
Physical Medicine & Rehabilitation	370	479	95%	58%	13	101	42	27
Neurology	581	704	97%	58%	14	45	41	152
Internal Medicine	4,922	7,697	98%	43%	84	306	470	1,335
Family Medicine	2,535	3,302	98%	44%	80	244	420	482

---

26 Statistics apply to *integrated* Thoracic Surgery, Vascular Surgery and Plastic Surgery. Integrated programs accept applicants from medical school, while fellowship programs accept applicants from a general surgery residency.

Table 16.3. *Data of applicants who successfully matched by specialty (28, 100-102)*

(Calculations include both U.S. Allopathic Seniors and Independent applicants)

Specialty	Average USMLE Step 1	Average USMLE Step 2	% US Seniors who were AOA	Average # Abstracts, Presentations and Publications
Plastic Surgery	242	242	42	9
Dermatology	240	248	51	7
Otolaryngology (ENT)	240	245	37	4
Neurosurgery	239	237	28	8
Radiation Oncology	238	241	35	8
Diagnostic Radiology	238	242	23	4
Orthopedic Surgery	237	240	28	4
Ophthalmology	235	-	-	-
Pathology	226	227	13	5
Neurology	225	229	12	4
Anesthesiology	224	230	10	2
Internal Medicine	224	229	15	3
General Surgery	224	230	12	3
Internal Medicine/Pediatrics	222	231	21	2
Child Neurology	221	-	-	-
Emergency Medicine	221	229	11	2
Pediatrics	218	227	12	2
Obstetrics & Gynecology	217	227	14	2
Physical Medicine & Rehabilitation	213	216	4	2
Psychiatry	213	217	4	2
Family Medicine	208	214	5	1

Do not let these statistics lead you to believe that all the best students go into Plastic Surgery and Dermatology. The number of outstanding students who go into the specialties of Internal Medicine and Pediatrics probably exceeds that of the smaller, more competitive specialties. It is the number of training positions available that primarily makes some specialties more competitive than others. The differences in the number of training positions among specialties, by and large, reflect the relative need of that specialty by society. For example, the United States needs far more internists than plastic surgeons because the ailments treated by internists are more prevalent than the ailments treated by plastic surgeons.

Competitive specialties have the luxury of being more selective, which elevates the average quality, or competiveness, of their residents. Let's assume the population of plastic surgery applicants is equivalent to the population of internal medicine applicants, that, in other words, the "bell-curves" of applicant quality are equivalent. In order to fill all of their training positions, internal medicine has to accept 98% of all applicants; therefore the quality or competitiveness of their residents is roughly equivalent to that of their applicants, because they had to accept applicants from both sides of the curve in order to fill all the training positions. Plastic surgery, on the other hand, has the luxury of only accepting the top 53% of applicants, or the top half of the curve. Therefore, those who match into plastic surgery will be more competitive as a group than those who match into internal medicine as a group. It is the ability to be more selective that explains why the average USMLE scores, percentage who are AOA, and research productivity are higher among those who match into plastic surgery than those who match into internal medicine.

Looking at match data is bittersweet. The bitter part is that not everyone matches into the specialty of his or her choice. Nearly half of the applicants who applied for plastic surgery training positions did not match in plastic surgery, and 30% of applicants who applied for dermatology training positions did not match in dermatology. The sweet part is that 98% of applicants for training positions in internal medicine, family medicine and pediatrics successfully matched. If you go to medical school, make it through, have an appreciation of how competitive an applicant you are and play the match game appropriately, a rewarding career awaits you.

After you submit your "rank list" to the NRMP and the deadline to make changes or withdraw from the match passes, you automatically enter into a binding contract with whichever program you matched with. This should not be a problem because you will only rank those programs where you are willing to train. This binding contract that becomes active when the rank order list deadline passes serves to protect programs and other applicants. Let's say you are a residency program director and you match your 3rd, 7th and 11th choices. Your 7th choice then changes their mind and breaks contract. This is unfair for the program, because if #7 had withdrawn before the match, the program might have ended up with their 3rd, 11th, and 14th choices, which is far better for them than having to scramble for an unmatched applicant. This is also unfair for other applicants, because #14 would have ended up at that program, but matched somewhere else or not at all. If #14 had matched there, then another applicant could have matched where #14 ended up matching, and so on. Withdrawing from a training position after the match has taken place is less than ideal for both programs and applicants, which is why there are consequences in place if you break contract and withdraw after the match.

Osteopathic residency training positions are available only to osteopathic medical students and graduates. There are not enough osteopathic residency training positions to accommodate all graduating osteopathic medical students. Many osteopathic seniors and graduates apply to both allopathic residencies and osteopathic residencies, and must therefore register with both the NRMP and the National Matching Services© (NMS). The Osteopathic Residency Match is administered by the National Matching Services (NMS) with oversight by the AOA (59). Osteopathic match results are released in early February. This gives successfully matched osteopathic applicants the ability to withdraw from the NRMP match before NRMP rank lists are due and contracts become binding.

Table 16.4. *Osteopathic Residency Match (103)*

	Positions	Filled
Anesthesiology	26	23
Dermatology	30	27
Emergency Medicine	210	201
Emergency Medicine/Internal Medicine	23	17
Family Practice	661	322
Family Practice/Emergency Medicine	10	10
General Surgery	98	86
Integrated Family Practice/Neuromusculoskeletal Medicine	9	7
Internal Medicine	415	241
Internal Medicine/Pediatrics	4	0
Neurological Surgery	15	13
Neurology	12	11
Neuromusculoskeletal Medicine/Osteopathic Manipulative Medicine	10	6
Obstetrics and Gynecology	64	56
Ophthalmology	11	10
Orthopedic Surgery	85	82
Otolaryngology & Facial Plastic Surgery	24	24
Pediatrics	62	45
Psychiatry	19	17
Traditional Rotating Internship (Transitional/Preliminary year)	642	263
Urological Surgery	8	7

Many osteopathic seniors seem to prefer allopathic residency programs as many osteopathic residency positions go unfilled despite the fact that there are fewer osteopathic residency training positions than there are osteopathic medical school graduates.

The Military Match takes place in December. All students who attend the Uniformed Services University or receive the Health Professions Scholarship from any of the three military branches are required to enter the military residency match and will likely train in a military sponsored residency program. Military residency training programs are ACGME accredited and therefore physicians are eligible for board certification in their specialty after completing these programs. If they do not match into one of the military residency programs, they will be authorized to apply for a civilian residency training position, which they will complete off active duty under a deferred status (45).

"Active Duty Training Programs" are military residency programs. While training in an active duty training program, residents are on active duty status and receive officer's basic pay, basic allowance for housing, basic allowance for subsistence and variable special pay (45). Active duty service obligations from college and medical school can be repaid concurrently during residency. Although residents accrue one year of active duty service obligation for each year they are in residency, they can repay previously accrued active duty service obligations during residency. For example, let's say you have 4 years of active duty service obligation from college, 4 years from medical school and you complete a 5-year residency at an active duty training program. Your total active duty service commitment is 13 years; however, you can repay 5 of those years concurrently with your active duty residency so that, after residency, you have an 8-year active duty service commitment.

Civilian Sponsored Training Programs are civilian residency programs sponsored by the military. Residents match into these positions through the military residency match. While training in a civilian sponsored training program, residents are on active duty status and receive officer basic pay, basic allowance for housing, basic allowance for subsistence and variable special pay (45). They will accrue one year of active duty service obligation for each year they are in residency. Previously accrued active duty service obligations cannot be repaid concurrently while attending civilian sponsored training programs.

Deferred Status is when the military allows one to spend time off active duty in order to obtain residency training in a civilian program. This is sometimes referred to as the DELAY program. Residents in deferred status defer their active duty obligations and do not receive any pay or benefits from the military (45). Upon completion of residency, they will return to active duty and complete their service requirement. Under deferred status, one does not accrue any active duty service obligations during residency unless they utilize the financial assistance program (FAP), which is outlined in chapter 5.

Depending on what you want to specialize in and where you want to train, being obligated to complete a military residency may put you at a disadvantage. Let's say you attend medical school under the Air Force HPSP, which obligates you to enter into the military match unless the military grants you deferment. You decide you want to be an orthopedic surgeon; however, there are not many orthopedic surgery training positions in the Air Force in your senior year. Because of this, the Air Force grants you deferment for 3 years. This isn't ultimately helpful, because you need 5 years to complete a civilian orthopedic surgery program. Ultimately, you could be forced to specialize in something else. The military will probably do their best to accommodate your career goals, but they have an obligation to create the physician workforce that the military needs.

Each year the Health Professions Education Requirement Board (HPERB) meets and decides the number of residency training positions in each specialty that will be available to that year's senior medical students. The number of training positions in each specialty is adjusted on an annual basis to reflect the needs of each military branch. The match is done by the Joint Service Graduate Medical Education Selection Board (JSGMEB).

Applications for military residency positions are submitted in September of the fourth year of medical school. The JSGMEB meets in late November and decides where each applicant will be receiving their residency training. The fate of each applicant is based on the applicant's rank list, the residency programs' rank lists and the applicant's "points" on the JSGMEB point scale (45).

Table 16.5. *Military Match (45)*

(Positions include Active Duty Programs and Civilian Sponsored Programs)

	Duration of Training Including Internship (years)	Positions in 2009 Air Force Match	Positions in 2007 Army Match	Positions in 2006 Navy Match
Aerospace Medicine	3	21	2	17
Anesthesiology	4	8	12	18
Dermatology	4	5	7	7
Diagnostic Radiology	5	16	15	15
Emergency Medicine	3	15	26	18
Family Medicine	3	44	43	44
Family Medicine/Aerospace medicine	5	5	0	0
General Preventative Medicine	3	9	0	0
General Surgery	5	16	29	10
Internal Medicine	3	42	50	32
Neurology	4	2	5	2
Neurosurgery	7	1	0	1
Obstetrics & Gynecology	4	9	15	13
Occupational Medicine	3	5	0	0
Ophthalmology	4	4	7	4
Orthopedic Surgery	5	4	19	11
Otolaryngology (ENT)	5	4	6	4
Pathology	4	3	6	5
Pediatric Neurology	4	0	1	0

	Duration of Training Including Internship (years)	Positions in 2009 Air Force Match	Positions in 2007 Army Match	Positions in 2006 Navy Match
Pediatrics	3	25	26	21
Preventative/Occupational Medicine	3	0	3	2
Psychiatry	4	13	14	12
Psychiatry/Internal Medicine	4	0	2	0
Radiation Oncology	4	2	1	0
Urology	6	2	0	2

17   Succeeding in the Residency Match

Your success in the residency match will largely depend on the strength of your application, which is determined by your accomplishments and performance in medical school. However, regardless of how stellar your application may be, playing the match game effectively is important to maximize your chances of success.

To maximize your chances of matching you need to apply to and interview at multiple programs of varying levels of competitiveness. In general, only programs that interview you will rank you, so you can only rank programs you interview at. In order to maximize your number of interviews, you need to apply to multiple programs. You cannot assume you will be offered an interview at every program you apply to, and you cannot assume that you will be able to schedule an interview at every program that offers you an interview. Let's say you are a superstar applicant, so you only apply to 5 programs. Four of these programs offer you interviews, but due to scheduling conflicts you can only attend 2 interviews. Therefore, you can only rank 2 programs in the match. Not only should you apply to many programs, but you should also diversify. Apply to some top-notch programs, apply to some average programs and apply to some "safety" programs. The beauty of the matching process is that you have nothing to lose by ranking a top-notch program #1, because if you don't match there you will just fall down to your #2 choice, which is where you would have started anyways if you hadn't put the top-notch program as #1.

ERAS will charge you more to apply to 30 programs than to 10 programs. It will cost you more to interview at 10 programs than at 5 programs. However, the cost of going unmatched will be much greater than the money you will save by only applying to and interviewing at a few programs. In 2009 the average matched applicant rank list had 9.4 programs on it (28).

Let's say you really want to be a dermatologist, but if you don't match into dermatology you would rather be a pediatrician than take a year off and risk not matching into dermatology again. In that case, it may be worthwhile to apply to, interview at and rank both dermatology and pediatrics programs. You can make your rank list such that dermatology programs are at the top and pediatrics programs are at the bottom. If you don't match into dermatology programs, hopefully a pediatrics program will pick you up before you fall to the bottom of your list and go unmatched.

Some medical students, especially those applying to competitive specialties, will do externships or "away rotations" at other institutions in the specialty they are interested in. These rotations must be scheduled months ahead of time and are usually about a month long. If you want to be an otolaryngologist (ENT) you will do an ENT rotation at your home institution and maybe one to two ENT rotations at other institutions. Doing away rotations will usually work to your advantage because it gives programs a chance to get to know you and gives you a chance to get to know that program. When program directors look at residency applications they try to figure out what an applicant is like and speculate how well they will fit in at their program. Doing an away rotation takes a lot of the figuring and speculation out of the equation and makes you a known entity. Doing an away rotation also shows the program your interest in their program. Finally, rotating at an outside institution will give you an opportunity to ask for letters of recommendation from faculty at that institution.

18   Subspecialty Match

Some will argue that it is premature for a pre-med or medical student to be thinking about sub-specialties – I disagree. Let's say you are a third year medical student on your internal medicine rotation and you realize that you love gastroenterology but don't particularly like internal medicine. Well, you should be aware that gastroenterology fellowships, which you enter after an internal medicine residency, have a 54% match rate. If you do well in residency, work hard, do some research, and so on, you should have a good chance of matching into a gastroenterology fellowship. However, if you don't match, which is a real possibility, you will be an internist, which is unfortunate if you don't particularly like internal medicine. Be careful about doing a residency in a specialty you don't particularly like, because there are no guarantees that you will get the fellowship you want.

Table 18.1. *Subspecialty Match (104, 105)*

Subspecialty	Applicants	Positions	Matched	Match Rate (%)
Internal Medicine				
Allergy & Immunology	174	115	108	62
Cardiology	1159	712	702	61
Clinical Oncology	191	44	40	21
Endocrinology	325	223	195	60
Gastroenterology	608	339	328	54
Hematology	124	22	21	17
Hematology & Oncology	706	426	413	58
Infectious Disease	331	303	267	81
Nephrology	578	367	348	60
Pulmonary Disease	86	20	20	23
Pulmonary Disease & Critical Care Medicine	607	397	387	64
Rheumatology	243	181	168	69

Subspecialty	Applicants	Positions	Matched	Match Rate (%)
Obstetrics & Gynecology				
Female Pelvic Medicine & Reconstructive Surgery	50	27	27	54
Gynecologic Oncology	73	47	44	60
Maternal-Fetal Medicine	135	87	83	61
Reproductive Endocrinology	70	39	38	54
Orthopedic Surgery				
Foot and Ankle Orthopedics	46	58	44	96
Hand Surgery	150	137	126	84
Orthopedic Foot & Ankle Surgery	47	62	38	81
Orthopedic Spine Surgery	133	122	97	73
Orthopedic Sports Medicine	241	224	184	76
Orthopedic Trauma Surgery	110	81	69	63
Otolaryngology				
Facial Plastic Surgery	63	43	43	68
Neurotology	28	11	11	39
Pediatric Otolaryngology	55	32	32	58
Rhinology	30	23	16	53
Pediatrics				
Allergy & Immunology	174	115	108	62
Neonatal-Perinatal Medicine	184	208	160	87
Pediatric Cardiology	163	108	104	64
Pediatric Critical Care Medicine	116	141	110	95
Pediatric Emergency Medicine	134	118	109	81
Pediatric Gastroenterology	82	60	56	68
Pediatric Hematology/Oncology	144	142	123	85
Pediatric Rheumatology	20	22	17	85
Pediatric Sports Medicine	28	12	12	43
Psychiatry				
Child & Adolescent Psychiatry	285	304	251	88
Diagnostic Radiology				
Interventional Radiology	109	185	99	91
Neuroradiology	145	190	127	88
General Surgery				
Abdominal Transplant Surgery	86	78	55	64

Subspecialty	Applicants	Positions	Matched	Match Rate (%)
Colon & Rectal Surgery	113	78	76	67
Hand Surgery	150	137	126	84
Pediatric Surgery	61	40	40	66
Plastic Surgery Fellowship	201	101	98	49
Surgical Critical Care	95	143	85	89
Thoracic Surgery	101	118	94	93
Vascular Surgery	113	116	102	90
Family Medicine				
Primary Care Sports Medicine	183	138	133	73
Urology				
Female Pelvic Medicine & Reconstructive Surgery	50	27	27	54
Plastic Surgery				
Craniofacial Surgery	46	23	19	41
Hand Surgery	150	137	126	84
Ophthalmology				
Occuloplastic Surgery	35	18	18	51
Neurology				
Neurocritical Care	31	49	25	81
Dermatology				
Mohs Micrographic Surgery	82	56	48	59
Pediatric Dermatology	16	20	13	81

19 Conclusion

The road to becoming a physician is a long, complicated and expensive one.

If you want to have 4 children before you are 30 years old, you may want to consider a career that doesn't require you to sacrifice so much of your time and youth.

If you want to be a millionaire by the time you are 40 years old, you may want to explore careers in another field.

If you only want to go to medical school so you can become a dermatologist, you may want to reconsider, because there are no guarantees that you will be one of the applicants who successfully matches into a dermatology residency.

If you still want to be a physician now that you are informed of the risks, benefits and alternatives – then go for it because it may be one of the best decisions you ever make.

Short of marrying my wife, the decision to go to medical school and become a physician was the best decision I have ever made. I am a better, happier and more fulfilled person because of it. The challenges of medical school gave me a much deeper and better understanding of myself and made me a more productive person. More importantly, medical school has given me knowledge and skills that enable me to be of greater service to other people. There is nothing I would rather do with my life than serve others as a physician.

Whether you find your calling in medicine or not, I wish you the best in finding it.

Appendix 1   53 Careers in Healthcare – The Alternatives

Nearly all the careers available to you in the healthcare industry have a nationally standardized training process. Pharmacists all have to take the same college pre-requisite courses, the same entrance exam, and the same board exams. The same goes for physicians, podiatrists, nurse practitioners, physician assistants, dentists, etc. This chapter will give you an overview of the training process for 53 careers in healthcare.

Although not all healthcare careers are mentioned below, you can see that there are many careers in the healthcare industry - all of which serve others in some way. In addition to reading through the brief descriptions that follow, I encourage you to investigate the careers that interest you. Do some research online and contact your local hospital and make arrangements to spend the day with someone who does what you are interested in. While investigating different careers, consider how they will fit into your life. For example, if you want to live in a rural community and work at the local hospital - you probably will not be able to do so as an electroneurodiagnostic technologist.

You may be surprised by the disparity in income among different healthcare careers. Why does a nurse-anesthetist, who trained for the same amount of time as a pharmacist, make, on average, $50,000 more than a pharmacist? The primary reason is that healthcare is not a free market; the market does not naturally adjust incomes on the basis of supply and demand. Instead, incomes are primarily determined by the amount the government and insurance companies have decided to reimburse for each service. If you happen to provide a service for which your employer is generously reimbursed, your income is likely to be higher. If you provide a service for which there is a meager reimbursement, your income is likely to be lower.

Table A.1.   *Careers in Healthcare*

	Post-Secondary Training[27] (years)	Median Gross Income[28] (36, 37, 106-150)(30, 35, 151) ($)	Median Net Income[29] (91) ($)
Nurse's Assistant	0.04	27,141	25,065
Phlebotomist	0.06	25,000	23,088
Emergency Medical Technician	0.06	29,040	26,749
Pharmacy Technician	0.50	26,600	24,565
Paramedic	0.50	37,502	33,556
Medical Assistant	1.00	28,300	26,135
Dental Assistant	1.00	32,380	29,465
Licensed Practical Nurse	1.00	39,030	34,777
Optician	2.00	32,810	29,809
Dental Lab Technologist	2.00	34,170	30,895
Medical Laboratory Technician	2.00	35,380	31,861
Surgical Technologist	2.00	38,740	34,545
Histology Technician	2.00	40,000	35,507
Electroneurodiagnostic Technologist	2.00	46,351	40,139
Cardiovascular Technologist	2.00	47,010	40,618
Respiratory Therapist	2.00	52,200	44,389
Radiology Technologist	2.00	52,210	44,397
Diagnostic Medical Sonographer	2.00	61,980	51,456
Registered Nurse	2.00	62,450	51,787
Dental Hygienist	2.00	66,570	54,691
Nuclear Medicine Technologist	2.00	66,660	54,712
Radiation Therapist	2.00	72,910	59,159
Child Life Specialist	4.00	39,000	34,753
Athletic Trainer	4.00	39,640	35,237
Kinesiotherapist	4.00	40,000	35,507
Dietician	4.00	50,590	43,219
Medical Laboratory Technologist	4.00	53,500	45,334
Perfusionist	4.00	111,006	83,329

[27]   Refers to the most direct and most typical pathway if one attends school full-time.

[28]   "Gross income" refers to one's income before taxation. "Median" means that 50% earn more and 50% earn less than the amount listed.

[29]   Calculated based on 2010 income tax rates for someone living in California, married with two children and opting out of the California state disability insurance. Calculation performed at www.paycheckcity.com. Federal income tax varies with gross income (see Tables 6.1 and 6.2). The California 2010 state personal income tax rate is 6.6%.

	Post-Secondary Training[27] (years)	Median Gross Income[28] (36, 37, 106-150)(30, 35, 151) ($)	Median Net Income[29] (91) ($)
Molecular Genetics Technologist	5.00	54,000	45,698
Cytogenetic Technologist	5.00	54,072	45,750
Genetic Counselor	5.50	62,852	52,071
Occupational Therapist	5.50	66,780	54,839
Public Health Worker	6.00	55,000	46,424
Prosthetist/Orthotist	6.00	67,078	55,049
Physical Therapist	6.00	72,790	59,074
Anesthesiology Assistant	6.00	81,200	64,989
Clinical Nurse Specialist	6.00	85,613	68,002
Nurse Midwife	6.00	90,010	71,004
Social Worker	6.50	46,650	40,356
Speech and Language Pathologist	6.50	62,930	52,125
Physician Assistant	6.50	85,710	68,068
Licensed Professional Counselor	7.00	35,451	31,918
Chiropractor	7.00	66,490	54,634
Nurse Practitioner	7.00	87,575	69,431
Pharmacist	7.00	106,410	80,503
Nurse Anesthetist	7.00	153,921	109,832
Marriage & Family Therapist	8.00	44,590	38,859
Optometrist	8.00	175,329	122,858
Dentist	8.00	220,000	149,681
Audiology	9.00	62,030	51,491
Dentist – Endodontist	10.20	394,120	246,105
Clinical Psychologist	11.00	64,140	52,978
Podiatrist	11.00	113,650	84,943
Physician – Family Medicine	11.00	197,655	136,264
Physician – Pediatrics	11.00	202,832	139,372
Physician – Internal Medicine	11.00	205,441	140,939
Physician – Obstetrics & Gynecology	12.00	294,190	191,099
Physician & Dentist - Oral Surgery	14.00	400,000	249,262
Physician – Neurosurgery	15.00	548,186	327,867

Nurse's Assistant (C.N.A.)

Certified Nurse Assistant
Also known as: Nurse's aide, Nursing assistant

Description

Nurse's assistants care for patients under the supervision of nurses and physicians. They help patients with the activities of daily living such as eating, bathing, dressing and transferring in and out of bed.

Training

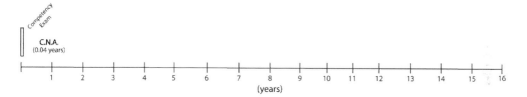

To become a nurse's assistant, one must complete a minimum of 75-hours of state-approved training. Some states require up to 150 hours of training. After passing a competency exam nurse's assistants become certified (C.N.A.) and are placed on the state registry of nurse's aides.

Median Gross Income: $27,141 (106)

Informative Websites

www.nahcacares.org
www.cna-network.org

Phlebotomist (C.P.T. or R.P.T.)

Certified Phlebotomy Technician, Registered Phlebotomy Technician

Description

Phlebotomists collect blood samples from patients via venupuncture.[30] They are trained to use the appropriate collection devices and transport medium for the test(s) ordered.

Training

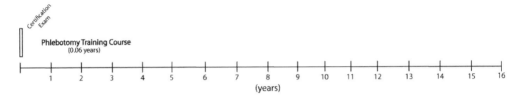

To become a phlebotomist one must complete a phlebotomy training course, which is about 120 hours, or 3 weeks, long. After successfully completing a training course, one may become certified/registered by the American Society for Clinical Pathology (ASCP), the American Medical Technologists (AMT) or the American Society for Phlebotomy Technicians (ASPT).

Median Gross Income: $25,000 (107)

Informative Websites

ww.aspt.org
www.nationalphlebotomy.org

---

[30]   Insertion of a needle into a vein

Emergency Medical Technician (EMT-B, EMT-I/85, EMT-I/99, EMT-P)

EMT-Basic, EMT-Intermediate, EMT-Paramedic

Description

Emergency medical technicians care for and transport the injured and ill to a medical facility. They work closely with firefighters and police officers. EMTs assess patients and provide emergency medical care as per the protocols provided by a physician medical director. On arrival at the emergency department, EMTs report the patient's history, their observations on the scene and interventions they provided en route.

The basic level of EMT (EMT-B) is trained to assess patients and manage respiratory, cardiac and trauma emergencies. EMT-Bs perform basic airway management, administer oxygen, give artificial respirations, perform CPR and defibrillate using an AED. EMT-Bs are also trained to take vital signs, perform spinal immobilization, bandage wounds, splint fractures and administer nitrogylcerin, glucose, epinephrine, and albuterol as per protocol.

The 1985 intermediate level EMTs (EMT-I/85) have additional training in IV therapy and multi-lumen airway management.

The 1999 intermediate level EMTs (EMT – I/99) have additional training in cardiac monitoring and medication administration.

Paramedics (EMT-P) have the most training among EMTs. They are trained to perform endotracheal intubation, place intravenous lines, and administer a variety of medications as per the medical director's protocol. Paramedics are trained to interpret electrocardiograms and defibrillate patients as per Advanced Cardiac Life Support (ACLS) algorithms.

Flight medics care for patients while they are being transported to a medical facility by helicopter. Flight medics are usually paramedics who have several years of experience. Flight nurses also care for patients while they are being transported to a medical facility.

Training

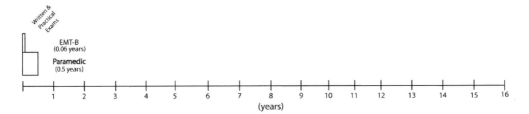

The National Registry of Emergency Medical Technicians (NREMT) is a private organization that certifies five levels of emergency medical service providers. Each level of NREMT certification requires the completion of the respective training requirements and passing a cognitive (written) and psychomotor (practical) examination. These examinations meet the National Highway Traffic Safety Administration's (NHTSA) standards.

First Responder ~40 hours of training
EMT – Basic ~110 hours (3 weeks) of training
EMT – Intermediate/85 ~200 hours (5 weeks) of training
EMT – Intermediate/99 ~400 hours (10 weeks) of training
EMT – Paramedic ~1,000 hours (6 months) of training
EMT-B Median Gross Income: $29,040 (108)
EMT-P Median Gross Income: $37,502 (152)

Informative Websites

www.naemt.org
www.nremt.org

Pharmacy Technician (C.Ph.T.)

Certified Pharmacy Technician

Description

Pharmacy technicians assist licensed pharmacists. They receive prescription requests, count tablets and label bottles. Pharmacy technicians may also perform administrative duties and provide customer service. In healthcare facilities, pharmacy technicians may prepare sterile solutions and deliver medications.

Training

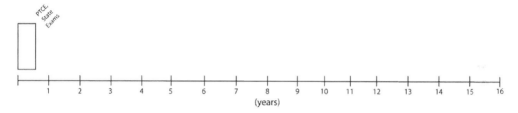

There are no standard training requirements for pharmacy technicians. Some states require pharmacy technicians to become licensed and/or registered by passing a state examination. Pharmacy technicians can become certified by the Pharmacy Technician Certification Board after passing the Pharmacy Technician Certification Exam (PTCE). One must hold a high school diploma or GED to be eligible to take the PTCE. Formal training programs are available at community and technical colleges. These programs are from 6 months to 2 years in length.

Median Gross Income: $26,600 (110)

Informative Websites

www.ptcb.org
www.nationaltechexam.org
www.ashp.org
www.pharmacytechnician.org

Medical Assistant (C.M.A.)

Certified Medical Assistant

Description

Medical Assistants are specifically trained to work in clinics. They perform administrative tasks such as answering telephones, scheduling appointments, updating medical records, filling out insurance forms, setting up diagnostic tests and arranging for hospital admissions. Medical assistants also perform clinical tasks such as taking vital signs, collecting laboratory specimens, sterilizing medical instruments, removing sutures, changing dressings, preparing patients for examinations and assisting physicians during examinations.

Training

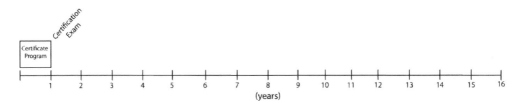

Both one-year certificate programs and two-year associate's degree programs exist. The Commission on Accreditation of Allied Health Education Programs (CAAHEP) or the Accrediting Bureau of Health Education Schools (ABHES) accredits training programs. To become certified, one must pass the CMA certification exam administered by the Certifying Board of the American Association of Medical Assistants.

Median Gross Income: $28,300 (127)

Informative Websites

www.aama-ntl.org

118

Dental Assistant (C.D.A.)

Certified Dental Assistant

Description

Dental assistants work under the supervision of dentists. They update patient's dental records, disinfect instruments and equipment, prepare instruments, equipment and materials for procedures and assist dentists during procedures.

Training

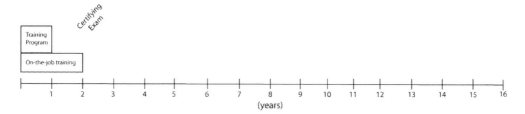

Most programs are one year long and lead to a certificate or diploma. Some community and technical colleges offer two year programs which lead to an associate degree. The Commission on Dental Accreditation (CODA) accredits dental assistant programs. Dental assistants can become certified by passing the Dental Assisting National Board (DANB) exam. To be eligible for examination, candidates must have graduated from an accredited dental assisting program or have two years of full-time on the job training.

Median Gross Income: $32,380 (133)

Informative Websites

www.danb.org
www.dentalassistant.org

119

Licensed Practical Nurse (L.P.N.)

Also known as: Licensed Vocational Nurse (L.V.N.)

Description

LPNs care for patients under the direction of physicians and registered nurses (RNs). LPNs provide basic bedside care to patients. They may supervise nursing assistants and aides. LPNs may collect samples for laboratory testing and assist physicians with procedures. In some states, LPNs are permitted to start intravenous fluids and administer prescribed medications.

Training

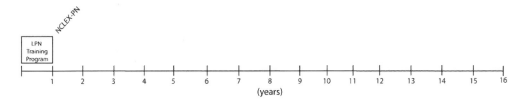

Most LPN training programs are one-year long. These programs are offered at community and technical colleges. To obtain licensure as an LPN, one must pass the NCLEX-PN.

Median Gross Income: $39,030 (128)

Informative Websites

www.napnes.org
www.nflpn.org
www.nln.org
www.ncsbn.org

Optician

Also known as: Dispensing optician

Description

Opticians help people select eyeglasses and fit them to their face. When helping customers choose eyeglasses, dispensing opticians consider the customer's occupation, hobbies and facial features. Opticians prepare work orders for ophthalmic laboratory technicians who fabricate and insert lenses into frames. Opticians also dispense contact lenses.

Opticians should not be confused with optometrists (O.D.) who examine patient's eyes and prescribe eyeglasses and contacts or ophthalmologists (M.D.) who perform surgery on the eyes.

Training

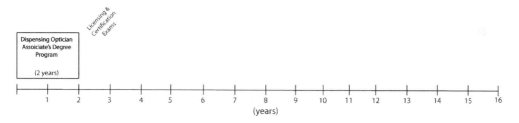

In some states anyone with a high school diploma can work as an optician. However, most employers, regardless of what state they are in, prefer opticians who have completed formal training and are licensed. Formal training is offered at community and technical colleges through a two-year associate's degree program. Licensing varies by state. Some states have their own written and practical exams. However, most states honor the certification exams offered by the American Board of Opticianry (ABO) and the National Contact Lens Examiners (NCLE). Anyone who is 18 years old and has a high school diploma is eligible to sit for these exams and become licensed.

Median Gross Income: $32,810 (123)

Informative Websites

www.oaa.org
www.abo.org
www.abo-ncle.org
www.nfos.org

Dental Laboratory Technician (C.D.T.)

Certified Dental Technician

Description

Dental laboratory technicians make dental prosthetics such as crowns, bridges and dentures from the molds, casts and photos sent to them by dentists. Their work requires the use of small instruments and an artistic aptitude.

Training

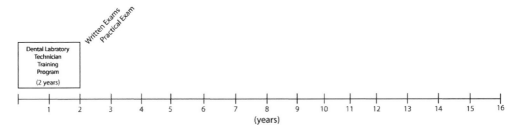

Most dental laboratory technician training programs are two years long. The Commission on Dental Accreditation (CODA) accredits dental lab technician training programs. After completing an accredited training program or five years of on-the-job training, dental lab technicians may become certified by successfully passing two written examinations and a practical exam offered by the National Board for Certification in Dental Laboratory Technology.

Median Gross Income: $34,170 (126)

Informative Websites

www.ada.org/profled/accred/commission/index.asp
www.ada.org/public/careers/team/lab.asp
www.nbccert.org

Medical Laboratory Technician (M.L.T.)

Also known as: Clinical Laboratory Technician

Description

Medical laboratory technicians prepare specimens and operate automated analyzers in medical laboratories. They usually work under the supervision of Medical Laboratory Technologists or laboratory managers. Technicians may become technologists through additional training.

Training

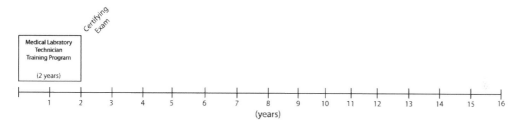

Medical laboratory technicians earn a two-year associates degree. The National Accrediting Agency for Clinical Laboratory Sciences (NAACLS) accredits medical laboratory technician training programs. Technicians may become certified by the American Society for Clinical Pathology (ASCP) or by the American Medical Technologist (AMT) by passing a certification exam.

Median Gross Income: $35,380 (107)

Informative Websites

www.alliedhealthschools.com/faqs/medical_lab_tech.php

Surgical Technologist (C.S.T.)

Certified Surgical Technologist
Also known as: Surgical Tech, OR Tech, Scrub

Description

Surgical technologists are members of the operating room team who assist surgeons in operations. They prepare the operating room by setting up surgical equipment and instruments. Surgical technologists pass instruments to surgeons while they operate. They may hold retractors, cut sutures, count sponges and prepare specimens for pathologic analysis.

With additional training, surgical technologists can become certified first assistants (CFA) or certified surgical assistants (CSA). First assistants may help provide exposure, achieve hemostasis and perform other technical maneuvers to help the surgeon.

Training

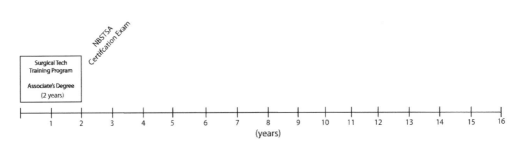

To become a surgical technologist, one must complete a training program that may last from 9 months to 2 years. Two-year programs usually award an associate's degree. Surgical technologist training programs are accredited by the Commission on Accreditation of Allied Health Education Programs (CAAHEP). To become certified, surgical technologists must pass a national certification exam offered by the National Board of Surgical Technology and Surgical Assisting (NBSTSA).

Median Gross Income: $38,740 (111)

Informative Websites

www.ast.org
www.lcc-st.org
www.nbstsa.org

Histology Technician (H.T.)

Also known as: Histotechnician

Description

Histotechnicans prepare tissue specimens for examination by pathologists. This preparation may involve the embedding, freezing, dehydrating, fixating, cutting, mounting and staining of tissue specimens.

Training

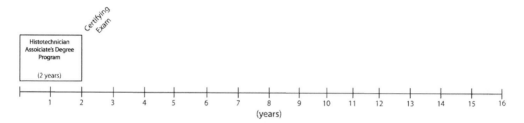

Histotechnician (H.T.) training programs are 12 months long, which may be part of an associate degree. Histotechnicians may become certified by the American Society for Clinical Pathology (ASCP) after passing a certification exam.

Median Gross Income: $40,000 (107)

Electroneurodiagnostic Technologist (R. EEG T., R. EP T., CLTM and CNIM)

Description

Electroneurodiagnistic technologists record, monitor, and analyze electrical activity arising from the brain, spinal cord and peripheral nerves. Tests they are trained to perform include the electroencephalogram (EEG), Nerve Conduction Studies (NCS), Evoked Potential studies (EP), intraoperaive neuromonitoring (IONP), Long Term Monitoring (LTM) and Polysomnograms (PSG).

Training

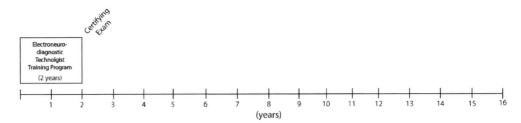

Most electroneurodiagnostic training programs are two-years long and award an associate's degree. The Commission on Accreditation of Allied Health Education Programs accredits Electroneurodiagnostic training programs. To become registered, electroneurodiagnostic technologists take registration exams offered by the American Board of Registration of Electroencephalographic and Evoked Potential Technologists (ABRET).

Median Gross Income: $46,351 (139)

Informative Websites

www.aset.org
www.aaet.info

Cardiovascular Technologist

Description

Cardiovascular technologists assist physicians in diagnosing and treating diseases of the heart and vascular system. They may specialize in invasive cardiology where they assist interventional cardiologists with cardiac catheterization procedures. Cardiovascular technologists may also specialize in non-invasive cardiology where they perform non-invasive diagnostic tests such as exercise stress tests and echocardiograms.

Training

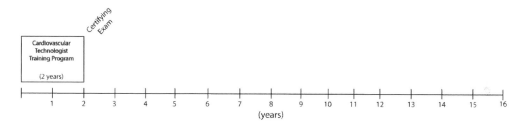

Cardiovascular technologists earn a 2-year associates degree. The first year consists of basic courses, the second year consists of instruction focused to their area of future specialization, invasive or non-invasive. The Commission on Accreditation of Allied Health Professionals (CAAHEP) accredits cardiovascular technologist programs. After completing an accredited program, Cardiovascular Technologists take a credentialing exam offered by the Cardiovascular Credentialing International (CCI) or American Registry of Diagnostic Medical Sonographers (ARDMS).

Median Gross Income: $47,010 (136)

Informative Websites

www.acp-online.com

Respiratory Therapist (R.R.T. or L.R.T.)

Registered Respiratory Therapist, Licensed Respiratory Therapist

Description

Respiratory therapists care for patients with breathing disorders such as asthma, chronic obstructive pulmonary disorder (COPD) and pneumonia. They also care for patients with normal lungs who are unable to breathe on their own due to diseases of or injury to another organ system. They work in many settings including: emergency departments, intensive care units, neonatal intensive care units, sleep laboratories, pulmonary function laboratories and inpatient wards. Under the direction of a licensed prescriber, respiratory therapists can set up mechanical ventilators, change ventilator settings, administer oxygen, administer aerosolized medications, draw arterial blood, suction out respiratory secretions, and give chest physiotherapy.

Training

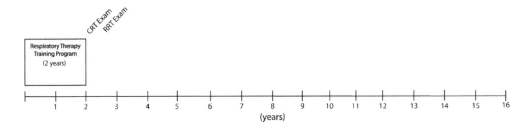

To become a respiratory therapist, one must earn an associate's degree in respiratory therapy. Respiratory therapy programs are accredited by the Committee on Accreditation for Respiratory Care (CoARC) or the Commission on Accreditation of Allied Health Education Programs (CAAHEP). To become a "registered" respiratory therapist, one must pass both the CRT and RRT exams offered by the National Board for Respiratory Care (NBRC).

Median Gross Income: $52,200 (114)

Informative Websites

www.aarc.org
www.caahep.org
www.nbrc.org

128

Radiology Technologist

Description

Radiology technologists perform diagnostic imaging of the body to help diagnose disease and injury. They operate X-ray machines, CT scanners, MRI machines and sonography equipment. Healthcare prescribers order diagnostic studies. Radiology technicians operate the equipment that generates images. Finally, radiologists and healthcare practitioners interpret the images.

Training

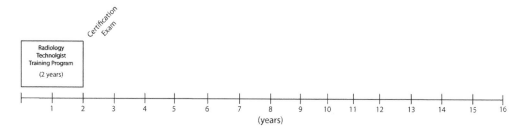

To become a radiology technologist, one must complete a certificate program, associate's degree program or bachelor's degree program. The most common route is the two-year associate's degree program. The Joint Review Committee on Education in Radiologic Technology accredits training programs in radiography. The American Registry of Radiologic Technologists (ARRT) offers certification for radiology technologists. In order to become licensed, most states require passing the respective ARRT certification exam.

Median Gross Income: $52,210 (115)

The AART provides certification in five primary disciplines of radiologic technology:

- Radiography (Radiology Technologist)
- Nuclear Medicine Technology
- Radiation Therapy
- Sonography
- Magnetic Resonance Imaging

After certification in one of the five primary disciplines, one may go on to become certified in the following specialties:

- Mammography
- Computed Tomography (CT)
- Magnetic Resonance Imaging (MRI)6

- Quality Management
- Bone Densitometry
- Cardiac-Interventional Radiography
- Vascular-Interventional Radiography
- Sonography[31]
- Vascular sonography
- Breast sonography

Informative Websites

www.asrt.org
www.jrcert.org
www.arrt.org

---

[31] Both primary and specialty tracks are available.

Diagnostic Medical Sonographer (R.D.M.S.)

Registered Diagnostic Medical Sonographer

Description

Sonographers use a transducer to deliver high frequency sound waves into patients' bodies. The return of these sound waves to the transducer creates images that are videotaped or photographed for interpretation by physicians. These images are used to diagnose and assess various diseases.

Training

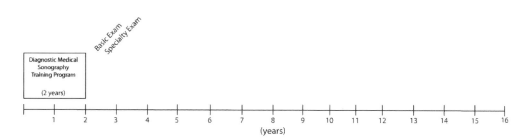

There are a number of paths one can take to become a sonographer. The most common path is a two-year associate's degree. Training programs are accredited by the Commission on Accreditation of Allied Health Education Programs (CAAHEP). People with an associate's degree in a patient-care allied health occupation can become eligible for certification after 12 months of full-time ultrasound experience. People with a bachelor's degree can become eligible for certification after 12 months of full-time ultrasound experience. Neither licensure nor certification is required to perform sonography; however, most employers prefer sonographers who are certified by the American Registry for Diagnostic Medical Sonography (A.R.D.M.S.). Certification involves passing a general exam and a specialty exam. Specialties include: abdomen, breast, obstetrics & gynecology, echocardiography, vascular technology, neurosonology, and ophthalmology.

Median Gross Income: $61,980 (130)

Informative Websites

www.sdms.org
www.ardms.org

Registered Nurse (R.N.)

Description

Registered Nurses comprise the largest and most diverse group within the healthcare occupations. In general, nurses provide more direct care and spend more time with a patient than any other healthcare provider. An internal medicine physician may round on over 30 hospitalized patients each day. The internist will talk with a patient, examine them, review vital signs, review recent diagnostic studies and ultimately write orders to change a patient's care as the physician deems necessary. The nurse, on the other hand, spends their entire shift carrying out the physician's orders and directly caring for the patient. If the patient's condition changes or there is a problem with the physician's orders, the nurse will contact the physician.

Registered nurses care for patients as per the orders of a licensed prescriber[32]. They make patients as comfortable as possible, educate patients, provide emotional support to patients and their families, place intravenous lines, administer medications, administer intravenous fluids, record their observations and contact physicians as needed.

Many opportunities are available to registered nurses. RNs can work in outpatient clinics, adult inpatient wards, pediatric inpatient wards, emergency departments, operating rooms, intensive care units, newborn nurseries, mental health units, hospice facilities and long-term care facilities, to name only a few. They can specialize in areas such as diabetes education, HIV/AIDS, wound/ostomy/incontinence, forensics or infection control. RNs can also take on administrative roles, such as a nurse-manager, or teaching roles, such as a nurse-educator. RNs can also provide home-health care services.

RNs may go on to become advanced practice nurses, such as a nurse practitioner, nurse anesthetist, nurse midwife or clinical nurse specialist.

Training

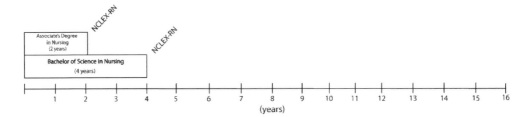

There are two major paths one can take to become a registered nurse, the associate's degree route and the bachelor's degree route. Two-year associate's degree programs

---

award an Associate's Degree in Nursing (A.D.N.). Four-year bachelor's degree programs award a Bachelor's of Science in Nursing (B.S.N.). In order to become a Licensed and Registered Nurse (R.N.), both ADNs and BSNs must pass the National Council Licensure Examination (NCLEX-RN). The National League of Nursing Accrediting Commission (NLNAC) and the Commission on Collegiate Nursing Education (CCNE) accredit nursing programs.

Which route should you take?

All of the advanced nursing degrees[33] are considered masters degrees, Master of Science in Nursing (M.S.N.). A bachelor's degree is a pre-requisite for admission into one of these master's degree programs. Moreover, a bachelor's degree is often necessary to take on nursing administration positions. If you think you may want to become a Nurse Anesthetist (C.R.N.A.), Nurse Practitioner (N.P.) or go into nursing administration, you should attend a nursing school where you can earn a Bachelors of Science in Nursing (B.S.N.). If you want to become an R.N. and have no aspirations of becoming an advanced practice nurse or taking on an administrative role, take the associate's degree route. If you change your mind later you can always attend an "R.N. to B.S.N. program." The title of these programs is misleading, as BSNs are Registered Nurses (R.N.) after they pass the NCLEX-RN. These programs should be titled "A.D.N. to B.S.N." Nonetheless, "R.N. to B.S.N." programs take about two years to complete, depending on the number of credits you start with and whether or not you attend school full-time. Some nursing schools offer one-year accelerated R.N. to B.S.N. programs for people who hold a bachelor's degree in another discipline.

Median Gross Income: $62,450 (37)

Informative Websites

www.nln.org
http://nursingworld.org
www.ncsbn.org
www.nacns.org
www.asrnorg

---

[33] Advanced Practice Nurses: Nurse Practitioner (N.P.), Certified Registered Nurse Anesthetist (C.R.N.A.), Certified Nurse Midwife (C.N.M.) or Clinical Nurse Specialist (C.N.S.)

Dental Hygienist (R.D.H.)

Registered Dental Hygienist

Description

Dental hygienists examine patients' mouths and remove plaque and other deposits from their teeth. Dental hygienists teach patients how to improve their oral hygiene and provide other types of preventative care.

Training

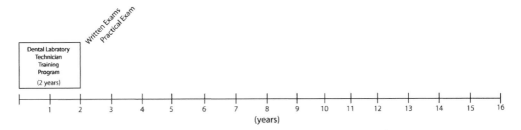

Most dental hygiene programs are two years long and lead to an associate's degree. 9.3% of programs offer a bachelor's degree in dental hygiene (153). Dental hygiene programs are accredited by the Commission on Dental Accreditation (CODA). After successfully completing a training program, dental hygienists must pass the Dental Hygiene National Board Exam administered by the American Dental Association's Joint Commission on National Dental Examinations.

Median Gross Income: $66,570 (132)

Informative Websites

www.adha.org

Nuclear Medicine Technologist (C.N.M.T.)

Certified Nuclear Medicine Technologist

Description

Radionuclides are unstable atoms that emit radiation spontaneously. Nuclear medicine utilizes radionuclides to detect disease by identifying metabolic changes. Nuclear medicine technologists administer radiopharmaceuticals to patients and operate gamma scintillation cameras that detect the radionuclide in the body. The images produced are then interpreted by physicians.

Training

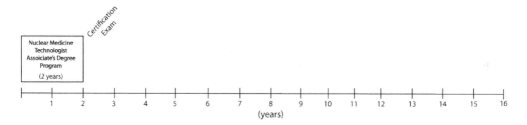

The most direct way to become a certified nuclear medicine technologist after high school is to earn an associate's degree from a community or technical college. 4-year bachelor's degree programs are also available. One-year certificate programs are available to health care professionals who have an associates or bachelor's degree in another discipline. Programs are accredited by the Joint Review Committee on Educational Programs in Nuclear Medicine Technology. Nuclear medicine technologists may become certified after passing an examination offered by the American Registry of Radiologic Technologists (ARRT) or the Nuclear Medicine Technology Certification Board (NMTCB).

Median Gross Income: $66,660 (125)

Informative Websites

www.snm.org
www.jrcnmt.org
www.arrt.org

Radiation Therapist

Description

Radiation therapy, or external beam radiation, is used to treat many types of cancer. Radiation therapists administer radiation to patients as prescribed by a radiation oncologist. They may help physicians localize the area requiring treatment via the use of fluoroscopy and CT scans.

Training

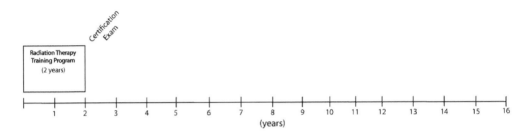

To become a radiation therapist, one must complete a two-year associate's degree program in radiation therapy. One-year certificate programs are available to those who already hold a degree in radiological imaging. The Joint Review Committee on Education in Radiologic Technology accredits radiation therapy training programs. The American Registry of Radiologic Technolgists (ARRT) offers certification for radiation therapists. In order to become licensed, most states require passing the respective ARRT certification exam.

Median Gross Income: $72,910 (116)

Informative Websites

www.arrt.org
www.asrt.org

136

Child Life Specialist

Description

Child life specialists prepare children for and support children through difficult tests and procedures. They help children cope with difficult situations through play, education and self-expression activities.

Training

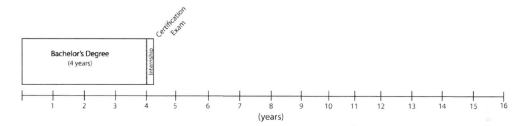

Child life specialists first earn a bachelor's degree in child life or a related field of study. To earn certification through the Child Life Council (CLC) they must complete a 480-hour internship and pass a certification exam. The internship is typically included in the curriculum of child life bachelor's degree programs.

Median Gross Income: $39,000 (140)

Informative Websites

www.childlife.org

Athletic Trainer

Description

Athletic trainers specialize in the prevention, assessment, diagnosis, treatment and rehabilitation of musculoskeletal injury and disease.

Training

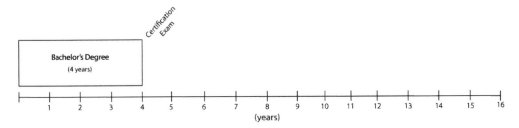

To become a certified athletic trainer one must earn a bachelor's degree from an accredited athletic training program and pass a certification exam. Training programs are accredited by the National Athletic Trainers' Association (NATA). The certification exam is offered by the Omaha based Board of Certification (BOC).

Median Gross Income: $39,640 (138)

Informative Websites

www.nata.org
www.bocatc.org

Kinesiotherapist

Description

Kinesiotherapists provide rehabilitation exercise and education to people with functional limitations and people who require physical conditioning. They apply scientifically based exercise principles to enhance the strength, endurance, mobility and flexibility of their clients.

Training

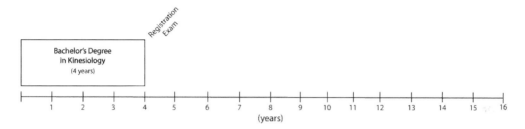

To become a kinesiotherapist, one typically earns a bachelor's degree in kinesiotherapy. Kinesiotherapy programs are accredited by the Committee on Accreditation of Allied Health Education Programs (CAAHEP). To become a registered kinesiotherapist, they must pass the Kinesiotherapy Registration Exam offered by the American Kinesiotherapy Association (AKA).

Median Gross Income: $40,000 (154)

Informative Websites

www.akta.org
www.caahep.org

Dietician (R.D.)

Registered Dietician

Description

Dieticians prevent illness and promote healing by recommending dietary modifications to patients and physicians. Dieticians assess a patient's nutritional needs, recommend a nutrition plan and evaluate the results.

Training

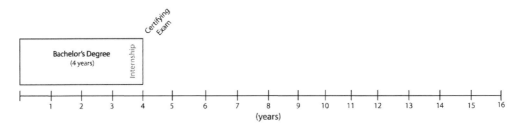

To become a registered dietician (R.D.) one must earn a bachelor's degree which meets the academic requirements set forth by the American Dietetic Association's (ADA) Commission on Accreditation for Dietetics Education (CADE). A 900-hour supervised internship must also be completed but may be integrated, or coordinated within, the bachelor's degree. Finally, dieticians must pass the registration examination for dieticians administered by the Commission on Dietetic Registration.

In most states, anyone can call them self a "nutritionist," as this does not imply any type of training or certification.

Median Gross Income: $50,590 (129)

Informative Websites

www.eatright.org
www.cdrnet.org

Medical Laboratory Technologist

Also known as: Clinical Laboratory Technologist, Medical Technologist, Clinical Laboratory Scientist

Description

Medical laboratory technologists work in medical laboratories where they perform chemical, biological, hematologic, immunologic, microscopic and bacteriologic tests.

Training

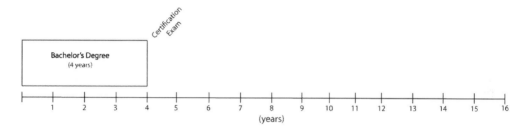

Medical laboratory technologists earn a bachelor's degree in medical technology or one of the life sciences. They may become certified by the American Society for Clinical Pathology, the American Medical Technologists, the National Credentialing Agency for Laboratory Personnel and/or the American Association of Bioanalysts.

Median Gross Income: $53,500 (107)

Informative Websites

www.acsls.org

Perfusionist (C.C.P.)

Certified Clinical Perfusionist

Description

Perfusionists operate extracorporeal circulation equipment such as heart-lung bypass machines and left ventricular assist devices. Perfusionists are responsible for the selection, setup and operation of this equipment. Extracorporeal circulation equipment is most commonly used during surgery on the heart and/or lungs.

Training

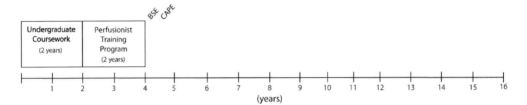

Perfusionist training programs are two years long. Some programs require two years of undergraduate coursework for admission and award a bachelors degree. Some programs require a bachelor's degree for admission and award a master's degree or a certificate. Perfusionist training programs are accredited by the Commission on Accreditation of Allied Health Education Programs. After completing an accredited training program, graduates are eligible for certification by the American Board of Cardiovascular Perfusion. To become certified, they must pass a basic science exam and the Clinical Applications in Perfusion (CAP) exam.

Median Gross Income: $111,006 (141)

Informative Websites

www.perfusion.com

Molecular Genetics Technologist

Description

Molecular genetics technologists study the relationship between genetics and disease. They extract DNA from tissues, perform polymerase chain reactions, gel electrophoresis, DNA & RNA sequencing and Southern blot analysis. Their work aids in the diagnosis, prognosis and monitoring of treatment.

Training

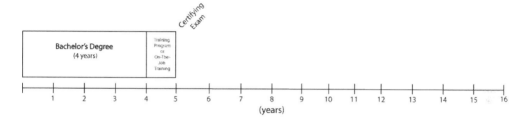

Molecular genetic technologists earn a bachelor's degree in a scientific discipline followed by a one-year molecular genetics training program or on-the-job training. They may become credentialed through the American Society for Clinical Pathology or the National Credentialing Agency.

Median Gross Income: $54,000 (142)

Cytogenetic Technologist

Description

Cytogenetic technologists study the morphology of chromosomes and how it relates to disease. They perform chromosomal staining, microscopic analysis, karyotyping and fluorescent in situ hybridization. Their work aids in the diagnosis, prognosis and monitoring of treatment.

Training

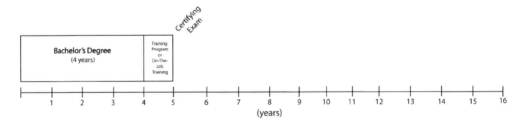

Cytogenetic technologists earn a bachelor's degree in a scientific discipline followed by a one-year cytogenetics training program or on-the-job training. They may become credentialed through the American Society for Clinical Pathology or the National Credentialing Agency.

Median Gross Income: $54,072 (143)

Genetic Counselor

Description

Genetic counselors support and educate patients and families who have genetic disorders or are at risk of having children with genetic disorders. They investigate heritable diseases present in the family and discuss available options with the family. Genetic counselors may specialize in prenatal, cancer, pediatric and adult.

Training

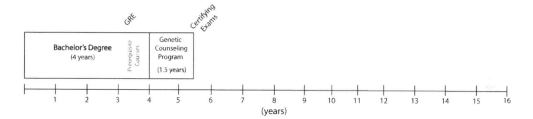

Genetic counselors must earn a master's degree in genetic counseling, be involved with 50 cases at an approved training site and pass both the general and specialty certification exams.

The American Board of Genetic Counseling (ABGC) certifies genetic counselors. Master's degree programs are typically around 18 months long. Requirements for admission include a bachelor's degree in biology, chemistry, psychology, social work, nursing, or another related field. Most programs also require applicants to take the GRE.

Median Gross Income: $62,852 (144)

Informative Websites

www.abgc.net
www.nsgc.org

Occupational Therapist (O.T.R.)

Occupational Therapist – Registered

Description

Occupational therapists help neurologically, physically and developmentally disabled people become more functional and more independent. Their treatments focus on improving function and compensating for permanently lost function. Occupational therapists often utilize adaptive equipment to help patients become more functional.

Training

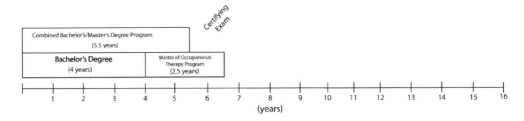

To become an occupational therapist one must earn a master's degree in occupational therapy. Combined bachelor's degree and master's degree programs are about five-and-a-half years long. Those with a bachelor's degree in another discipline can attend a master's degree program, which is about two-and-half years long. The Accreditation Council for Occupational Therapy Education (ACOTE) accredits occupational therapy programs. To become certified or "registered" one must pass the national certification exam offered by the National Board for Certifying Occupational Therapy.

Median Gross Income: $66,780 (124)

Informative Websites

www.aota.org

Public Health Worker (M.P.H)

Master of Public Health
Also known as: Public Health Professional

Description

Public health workers perform many different tasks and have diverse responsibilities. Public health workers are not trained to directly provide healthcare to patients, unless they have additional training as a physician, dentists, nurse, etc. Public health workers function at an administrative and political level to improve access to healthcare, minimize the spread of infectious disease, and reduce environmental hazards, substance abuse and violence. Public health workers serve at international, national, state and local levels. They may work as epidemiologists, policy analysts, food safety inspectors, health educators or researchers. Public health workers may work for the government, pharmaceutical companies, health insurance companies and non-profit organizations.

Training

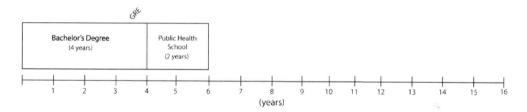

Public health workers come from many different educational backgrounds. Healthcare practitioners such as physicians and nurses often go on to earn a master's degree in public health. People with a bachelor's degree or higher can go on to earn a master's degree in public health (M.P.H.). These master's degree programs are typically about two years in length.

Median Gross Income (145):
Epidemiologist $68,000
Program Manager $52,071
Research Scientist: $50,000

Informative Websites

www.whatispublichealth.org
www.apha.org

Prosthetist/Orthotist (C.P.O.)

Certified Prosthetist and Orthotist

Description

Prosthetists and orthotists evaluate patients and then design, fabricate and fit orthoses and prostheses. Prostheses replace missing body parts. Orthoses support and/or correct the function of limbs.

Training

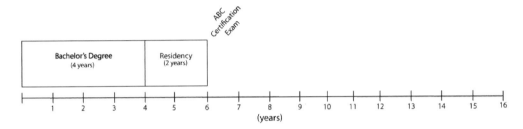

One can be trained and certified in orthotics, prosthetics or both. Certificate, bachelor's and master's degree programs are available. Orthotics and prosthetics training programs are accredited by the Commission on Accreditation for Allied Health Education (CAAHEP). After completing an accredited training program, one must complete a one-year residency in orthotics or prosthetics. To become certified in both orthotics and prosthetics, one must complete a one-year residency in each discipline. Residency programs are accredited by the National Commission on Orthotic and Prosthetic Education (NCOPE). To become certified by the American Board for Certification (ABC) in orthotics, prosthetics or both, one must complete an accredited training program, an accredited residency program and pass the respective certification exams.

Median Gross Income: $67,078 (146)

Informative Websites

www.ncope.org
www.abcop.org
www.opcareers.org
www.oandp.org
www.aopanet.org

Physical Therapist (P.T., L.P.T., R.P.T., D.P.T)

Physical Therapist, Licensed Physical Therapist, Registered Physical Therapist, Doctor of Physical Therapy

Description

Physical therapists treat patients whose movement and neuromusculoskeletal function is limited or threatened by disease, aging or injury. They help patients restore function, improve mobility, relieve pain and minimize permanent physical disabilities.

Training

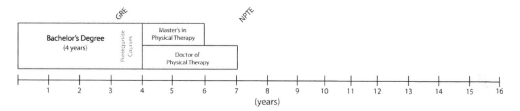

To become a physical therapist, one must earn a bachelor's degree and complete a two-year masters or three-year doctoral degree training program. Physical therapy training programs are accredited by the Commission on Accreditation of Physical Therapy Education (CAPTE). Licensing and registration requirements vary by state. However, most states require physical therapists to pass the National Physical Therapy Examination (NPTE).

Median Gross Income: $72,790 (120)

Informative Websites

www.apta.org

Anesthesia Assistant (AA-C)

Anesthesia Assistant - Certified
Also known as: Anesthesiology Assistant, Anesthesiologist Assistant

Description

Anesthesia Assistants administer anesthesia to patients during surgery under the direction of an Anesthesiologist. The Anesthesia Assistant independently monitors the patient and adjusts medications and fluids during the procedure. They are also trained in the management of both acute and chronic pain.

Training

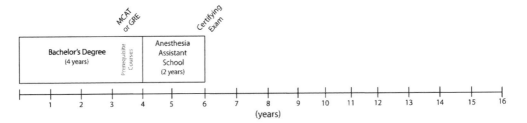

Anesthesia assistants first earn a bachelor's degree in any discipline and complete the required pre-requisite courses. Most programs require applicants to take the medical college admissions test (MCAT) or the GRE in order to be considered for admission. After completing a two-year training program accredited by the Committee on Accreditation of Allied Health Education Programs (CAAHEP), anesthesia assistants take the certifying examination for anesthesiologist assistants, which is administered by the National Commission for Certification of Anesthesiologist Assistants (NCCAA). After successfully passing this examination they may use the designation AA-C.

Median Gross Income: $81,200 (154)

Informative Websites

www.anesthetist.org
www.anesthesiaassistant.com
www.anesthesia-assistant.com

Clinical Nurse Specialist (C.N.S.)

Description

Clinical nurse specialists are advanced practice nurses who may work independently or in collaboration with physicians. Their prescriptive authority varies by state. Clinical nurse specialists may provide direct patient care and consultations in their nursing specialty. These nursing specialties include: acute care nursing, adult nursing, cardiovascular nursing, community health nursing, geriatric nursing, home health nursing, infectious disease nursing, neonatal nursing, occupational health nursing, oncology nursing, parent-child nursing, perinatal nursing, psychiatric nursing, rehabilitation nursing, school health nursing and women's health nursing. Clinical nurse specialists often have administrative roles where they work to improve patient outcomes by making changes to the hospital system and training nursing personnel.

Training

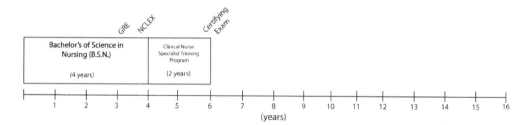

Clinical Nurse Specialists first earn a bachelors degree in nursing (B.S.N.) which takes 4 years. They then go on to earn a two-year masters degree in nursing (M.S.N.) during their clinical nurse specialist training. Some programs offer an RN to MSN path for registered nurses with an associate's degree; however, these programs are a couple of years longer. Some programs offer a direct entry MSN pathway for non-nurses who have a bachelor's degree in another discipline. Most programs require applicants to take the GRE in order to be considered for admission. Some programs also require several years of nursing experience to be considered for admission. Clinical nurse specialists may become certified by the American Nurses Credentialing Center (ANCC) after passing a specialty specific exam.

Median Gross Income: $85,613 (147)

Informative Websites

www.nacns.org
www.allnursingschools.com/faqs/cns.php

Nurse Midwife (C.N.M.)

Certified Nurse Midwife

Description

Nurse midwives are advanced practice nurses who are trained to deliver babies and provide prenatal and post-partum care to women. In most states, nurse midwives can prescribe medications. They may provide preventative healthcare and family planning services. Most nurse midwives focus their practice on caring for patients in labor and delivering babies. They are trained to recognize the signs and symptoms of a problem and know when to consult a physician. Nurse midwives are qualified to administer medications and perform procedures.

Training

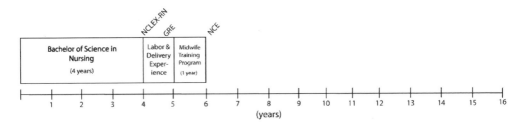

To become a nurse midwife one must first earn a bachelor's degree in nursing. There are a few programs that will accept applicants who have a bachelor's degree in another discipline. These individuals would then become certified midwives (C.M.). Most midwifery programs require at least one year of experience, preferably in labor and delivery. Most programs also require applicants to take the GRE. Nurse midwife training programs last one to two years. Nurse midwife training programs are master's degree programs that award a master of science in nursing (MSN). Midwifery training programs are accredited by the American College of Nurse-Midwives (ACNM) Accreditation Commission for Midwifery Education (ACME). To become certified, one must pass the national certification exam.

Median Gross Income: $90,010 (148)

Informative Websites

www.acnm.org
www.allnursingschools.com

Social Worker (L.C.S.W.)

Licensed Clinical Social Worker

Description

Social workers help people deal with crisis. Social workers in the healthcare setting provide psychosocial support to patients and their families to help them cope with illness and injury. One of the primary responsibilities of social workers in the healthcare setting is to arrange outpatient services, such as dialysis or home health care, for patients. While arranging these outpatient services, social workers must also find sources of funding for these services.

Training

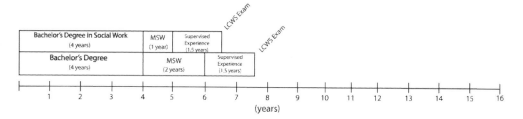

To become a licensed clinical social worker in the healthcare setting, one must earn a master's degree in social work (MSW), complete a supervised internship and pass the state-licensing exam. A master's degree in social work (MSW) is usually required to work in the healthcare setting. One can earn a master's degree in social work in about one year if one has a bachelor's degree in social work (BSW) or about two years if one has a bachelor's degree in another discipline. The Council on Social Work Education (CSWE) accredits master's degree programs in social work. After earning a master's degree, most states require the completion of 3,000 hours (1.5 years) of supervised clinical experience in order to be eligible for licensure. To become licensed, one must pass the licensing exams required by the state in which they wish to work.

Median Gross Income: $46,650 (113)

Informative Websites

www.socialworkers.org
www.centercsw.org
www.cswe.org
www.aswb.org

Speech and Language Pathologist (CCC-SLP)

Certificate of Clinical Competency in Speech and Language Pathology
Also known as: Speech Therapists

Description

Speech and language pathologists evaluate and diagnose speech disorders, language disorders, cognitive-communication disorders and swallowing disorders. They also provide therapy to treat people with these disorders.

Training

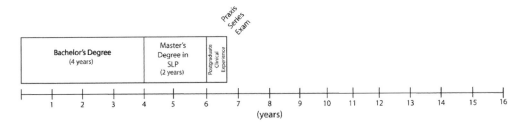

To become a speech and language pathologist certified by the American Speech-Language-Hearing Association (ASHA) one must earn a master's degree in speech and language pathology, complete a nine-month clinical fellowship and pass the Praxis Series examination in speech and language pathology. Master's degree programs are typically about two years in length. These programs are accredited by the American Speech-Language-Hearing Association's Council on Academic Accreditation. The requirements for earning the CCC-SLP credential outlined above meet licensure requirements in most states.

Median Gross Income: $62,930 (112)

Informative Websites

www.asha.org

Physician Assistant (P.A., PA-C)

Physician Assistant – Certified

Description

Physician assistants diagnose and treat patients under the supervision of a physician. They are trained to obtain a history, examine patients, order diagnostic studies and treat patients. Physician assistants can prescribe medications and perform small procedures as delegated to them by their supervising physician. Physician assistants work in all areas of medicine, from pediatrics to neurosurgery. Some physician assistants assist surgeons in the operating room.

Training

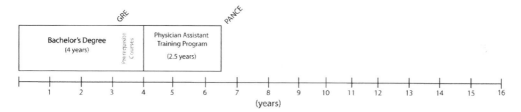

To become a physician assistant one must earn a bachelor's degree and complete a physician assistant training program. Physician assistant training programs are about two-and-a-half years long. These training programs are accredited by the Accreditation Review Commission on Education for the Physician Assistant (ARC-PA). Most of these programs award a master's degree at the time of graduation. To become certified, Physician Assistants must pass the Physician Assistant National Certifying Examination (PANCE) administered by the National Commission on Certification of Physician Assistants (NCCPA).

Table A.2.   *Admissions Data for the 2009 Incoming Physician Assistant Class[34] (155)*

Applicants	12,216
Training Positions	4,200
Acceptance Rate	34.4%
Avg. GPA among matriculants	3.46
Avg. GRE score among matriculants	1118

Median Gross Income: $85,710 (119)

---

[34]   Data is derived from the Central Application Service for Physician Assistants (CASPA), which is used by approximately 80% of U.S. Physicians Assistant training programs.

Informative Websites

www.aapa.org
www.arc-pa.org
www.nccpa.net
www.paeaonline.org

Licensed Professional Counselor (L.P.C.)

Also known as: Licensed Mental Health Counselor

Description

Licensed Professional Counselors provide individual and group psychotherapy. Their scope of practice varies by state. Licensed Professional Counselors cannot prescribe medications.

Training

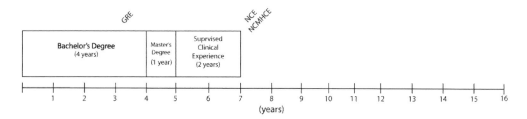

To become a Licensed Professional Counselor, one must first earn a master's degree in a related discipline such as psychology or social work. This is followed by two years of supervised clinical experience and licensing exams such as the National Counselor Examination for Licensure Certification (NCE) or the National Certified Mental Health Counselor Examination (NCMHCE).

Median Gross Income: $35,451 (149)

Informative Websites

www.counseling.org
www.guidetopsychology.com/cln_cns.htm

Chiropractor (D.C.)

Doctor of Chiropractic

Description

Chiropractors diagnose and treat patients with musculoskeletal problems and back pain. "Chiropractic" is based on the principle that spinal joint misalignments lower the human body's resistance to disease by interfering with the nervous system. Chiropractors cannot prescribe medications or perform surgery. Their treatments include manipulative therapy and teaching patients various exercises and remedies. Chiropractors may also provide health and lifestyle counseling.

Training

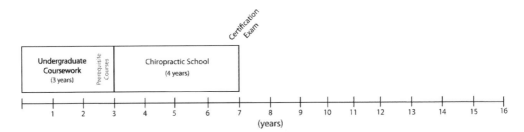

The amount of prior undergraduate coursework and pre-requisite courses vary among chiropractic schools; however, most schools require three years of undergraduate coursework including any pre-requisite courses. Most chiropractic colleges do not require applicants to take a standardized exam in order to be considered for admission (156). Chiropractors complete a 4-year training program at a Council on Chiropractic Education (CCE) accredited Chiropractic College. For licensure, most states accept the certification exam offered by the National Board of Chiropractic Examiners (NBCE).

Median Gross Income: $66,490 (135)

Informative Websites

www.acatoday.org
www.chiropractic.org
www.fclb.org
www.nbce.org
www.chirocolleges.org

Nurse Practitioner (N.P., NP-C)

Nurse Practitioner - Certified

Description

Nurse practitioners are advanced practice nurses who assess, diagnose, treat and manage the diseases and disorders that affect their patients. They assess patients by taking a history and performing a physical exam, and they may also order or perform diagnostic studies. Nurse practitioners can prescribe medications. Whether they may prescribe medications independently or only through collaboration with a physician varies by state.

Nurse practitioners specialize in a number of areas. The two-year NP curriculum focuses on one of these specialties and awards the respective credentials.

- Family (FNP)
- Adult (ANP)
- Pediatrics (PNP)
- Neonatology (NNP)
- Gerontology (GNP)
- Women's Health (WHNP)
- Psychiatry and Mental Health (PMHNP)
- Acute Care (ACNP)
- Oncology (ONP)

Training

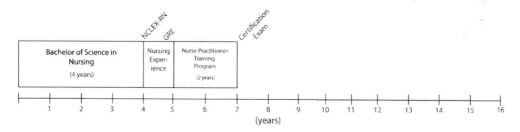

To become a nurse practitioner, one must first earn a bachelor's degree in nursing (BSN). Most NP training programs require at least one year of nursing experience in order to be considered for admission. There are, however, a few combined programs where the BSN and NP training are combined such that no time is spent working as an R.N. between nursing school and NP school. Most programs require applicants to take the GRE in order to be considered for admission. Nurse practitioner training programs are master's degree programs that award a master of science in nursing (MSN). Nurse practitioner training programs are accredited by the Commission on Collegiate Nursing

Education (CCNE) or the National League for Nursing Accrediting Commission (NLNAC). Nurse practitioners become certified in their specialty by passing the respective certification exam offered by the American Nurses Credentialing Center (ANCC).

Median Gross Income: $87,575 (150)

Informative Websites

www.aanp.org

Pharmacist (Pharm.D.)

Doctor of Pharmacy

Description

Pharmacists dispense prescription medications to patients that have been prescribed by licensed prescribers. Pharmacists cannot prescribe medications to patients. Pharmacists provide a layer of safety in patient care as they often catch errors made by prescribers, in which case they then contact the prescriber to clarify the dose. Pharmacists also help prescribers select the best medications and dosages for patients.

Training

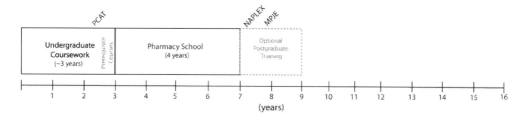

To become a pharmacist, one must complete two to four years of undergraduate coursework followed by four years of pharmacy school. Most pharmacy schools require applicants to take the Pharmacy College Admission Test (PCAT) in order to be considered for admission. Upon completion of pharmacy school, graduates are awarded a doctorate degree in pharmacy, Pharm.D. Historically, students earning a bachelor's degree in pharmacy were eligible to sit for the certification exams and become registered/certified; however, nowadays a Pharm.D. is required to become registered/certified in the United States. Pharmacy schools are accredited by the Accreditation Council for Pharmacy Education. To become licensed, all states require pharmacists to pass the North American Pharmacist Licensure Exam (NAPLEX). Most states also require pharmacists to pass the Multistate Pharmacy Jurisprudence Exam (MPJE).

Some pharmacists complete one or two year residencies in a specialty such as intravenous nutrition, oncology, critical care pharmacy, nuclear pharmacy, geriatric pharmacy and psychiatric pharmacy.

Median Gross Income: $106,410 (121)

Informative Websites

www.aacp.org
www.ashp.org
www.nacds.org
www.amcp.org
www.pharmacist.com
www.nabp.net
www.pcatweb.info
www.pharmcas.org

Nurse Anesthetist (C.R.N.A.)

Certified Registered Nurse Anesthetist

Description

Nurse anesthetists are advanced practice nurses who provide anesthesia to patients during surgery; they may also care for patients who suffer from chronic pain. Nurse anesthetists assess patients pre-operatively, administer anesthesia, intubate[35], monitor patients intra-operatively, maintain anesthesia intra-operatively and care for patients as they emerge from anesthesia. State law determines if nurse anesthetists can practice independently, without supervision or direction from an anesthesiologist.

Training

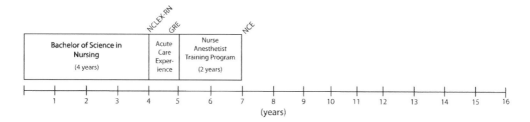

To become a Certified Registered Nurse Anesthetist (CRNA) one must first earn a bachelor's degree in nursing (BSN). Most nurse anesthetist training programs require at least one year of acute care nursing experience and a competitive GRE score in order to be considered for admission. Nurse anesthetist training programs are a minimum of two years long and award a masters degree in nursing (MSN). After graduating from an accredited training program, nurse anesthetists become certified by passing the National Certification Exam (NCE) offered by the Council on Certification of Nurse Anesthetists (CCNA).

Median Gross Income: $153,921 (151)

Informative Websites

www.aana.com
www.nbcrna.com

---

[35]   Insertion of an endotracheal tube into the trachea

Marriage and Family Therapist

Also known as: Marriage and Family Counselor

Description

Marriage and family therapists are trained in psychotherapy and family systems theory. They use this training to diagnose and treat mental disorders within the context of marriage, couples and family.

Training

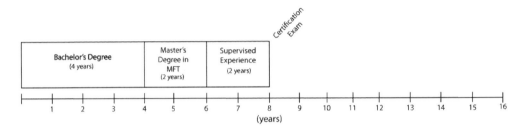

To become a licensed and certified marriage and family therapist, one must complete a master's degree program in marriage and family therapy, complete two years of supervised clinical experience, pass a national certification exam and pass any state licensing exams. Master's degree programs are about two years long. Training programs are accredited by the Commission on Accreditation for Marriage and Family Therapy Education (COAMFTE). A national certification exam is offered by the American Association for Marriage and Family Therapy (AAMFT). Some states require passing this certification exam in order to be eligible for licensure.

Median Gross Income: $44,590 (134)

Informative Websites

www.aamft.org
www.amftrb.org

Optometrist (O.D.)

Oculis Doctor
Also known as: Doctor of Optometry

Description

Optometrists examine patient's eyes and diagnose vision problems such as near-sightedness, far-sightedness, presbyopia, glaucoma and color blindness. When examining patient's retinas, optometrists may see signs of systemic disease such as diabetes or hypertension. Optometrists will then refer these patients to physicians for treatment of their systemic disease. Optometrists can prescribe refractive therapies in the form of eyeglasses and contacts. They can also provide vision therapy and low-vision rehabilitation. Optometrists can prescribe medications to treat diseases and disorders of the eye.

Training

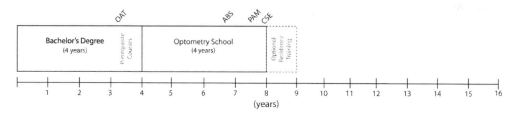

To become an optometrist, one must complete three years of bachelor's degree coursework followed by four years of training at an accredited college of optometry. 93% of students entering colleges of optometry in 2009 had a bachelor's degree (157). To be considered for admission, applicants must take the Optometry Admissions Test (OAT). The OAT consists of four sections: natural sciences (biology, chemistry, organic chemistry), reading comprehension, physics and quantitative reasoning. Applicants take the OAT one year before they hope to start optometry school as their score must be included in their application. Applications for optometry school are submitted via OptomCAS. Colleges of optometry are accredited by the Accreditation Council on Optometric Education of the American Optometric Association.

Table A.3.   *Colleges of Optometry 2009 Entering Class (157, 158)*

Applicants	2,822
Positions	1,665
Acceptance Rate	59%
Average Matriculant Undergraduate GPA	3.41
Average Matriculant OAT – Academic Average	335
Average Matriculant OAT – Total Science	340

To become licensed, optometrists must pass all three exams offered by the National Board of Examiners in Optometry (NBEO), Part 1, or the Applied Basic Science (ABS) exam, is taken in the spring of the third year of optometry school. Part 2, of the Patient Assessment and Management Exam (PAM) is taken in the middle of the fourth year of optometry school. Part 3, the Clinical Skills Exam (CSE) is taken near the end optometry school or after graduation.

One-year residency training programs are available to graduates of optometry school who wish to obtain further training in a particular area. These areas of specialization include: refractive & ocular surgery, cornea & contact lenses, low-vision rehabilitation, vision therapy & rehabilitation, ocular disease, community health optometry, primary eye care optometry, family practice optometry, pediatric optometry and geriatric optometry.

Mean annual income for self-employed optometrists in 2007: $175,329 (122)

Informative Websites

www.opted.org
www.aoa.org
www.optometry.org

Dentist (D.D.S. or D.M.D.)

Doctor of Dental Surgery, Doctor of Dental Medicine

Description

Dentists diagnose and treat diseases and disorders of the mouth. They extract teeth, fill dental carries, straighten teeth, repair fractured teeth and perform procedures to restore gums and supporting bones. Dentists are licensed to administer anesthetics and write prescriptions. General dentists frequently perform root canals, extract teeth, create crowns and bridges, place implants, construct dentures, treat gum disease and screen for oral cancer.

Training

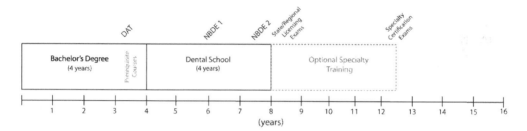

To become a dentist one must earn a bachelor's degree and graduate from dental school. Dental school is four years long. Roughly one fourth of dental school graduates pursue specialty training after dental school, which can take from one to four-and-a-half years. Many dental schools require only two-years of undergraduate coursework; however, 88.8% of first year dental students in 2008 had a bachelors degree and 6.2% had a master's or doctoral degree (159). Nearly all dental schools require pre-requisite courses in chemistry, physics, biology and organic chemistry. Applications to dental schools are submitted via the Associated American Dental Schools Application Service (AADSAS). Factors used to evaluate applicants for admission include undergraduate GPA, Dental Admissions Test (DAT) scores, letters of recommendation, community service, experience in the field and interviews by faculty. Nineteen dental schools in the U.S. offer a combined pre-dental/dental program in which students are offered admission after high school (15).

The DAT is a four and a half hour test consisting of 280 multiple choice questions (160). The exam is administered at Prometric™ testing centers. DAT scores are based on the number of correct responses; there is no penalty for guessing. Standard scores, ranging from 1 to 30, are reported to dental schools.

Table A.4. *Dental Admissions Test (DAT) (160)*

	Time (minutes)	Questions
Natural Sciences	90	100
Biology		40
General Chemistry		30
Organic Chemistry		30
Perceptual Ability	60	90
Apertures		
View Recognition		
Angle Discrimination		
Paper Folding		
Cube Counting		
3D Form Development		
Optional Break	15	
Reading Comprehension	60	50
Quantitative Reasoning	45	40

Table A.5. *Dental School Admission Information – 2008 Incoming Class (15, 159)*

Applicants	12,178
Matriculants	4,918
Matriculation Rate	40.4%
Average Matriculant DAT Scores	
Academic Average	18.8
Perceptual Ability	19.2
Total Science	18.9
Average Matriculant Science GPA	3.48
Average Matriculant Undergraduate GPA	3.54

Table A.6. *Average total cost of tuition & fees for all four years (15)*

In-state-resident at Public University	$115,988
In-state-resident at Private University	$208,597
Non-resident at Public University	$201,704
Non-resident at Private University	$215,611

Dental schools are accredited by the American Dental Association's Commission on Dental Accreditation (CODA). Approximately 96% of students who start dental school will graduate (15). Upon successful graduation from an accredited dental school, dentists are awarded the credentials of Doctor of Dental Surgery (D.D.S.) or Doctor of Dental Medicine (D.M.D.).

To become licensed and certified, dentists must pass both parts of the national certification exam as well as state or regional licensing exams. The National Board of Dental Examiners (NBDE) administers both parts of the national certification exam. Part one, or NBDE 1, is taken after the second year of dental school. NBDE 1 is a 7 hour, 400 question test that covers general anatomy, biochemistry, physiology, microbiology, pathology, dental anatomy and dental occlusion. NBDE 2 is taken during the fourth year of dental school. NBDE 2 is a 10.5 hour, 500 question test given over two days that covers operative dentistry, pharmacology, endodontics, peridontics, prosthodontics, orthodontics, oral surgery, pediatric dentistry, oral diagnosis, pain management and some basic sciences. State and regional licensing exams typically consist of a written and clinical component. These exams are taken at the end of dental school or shortly thereafter. 99.4% of the class of 2007 passed the national board exams and 98.3% passed their clinical licensure exams (159).

About a quarter of dental school graduates go on to receive specialty training, also known as advanced dental education. 1,670 students from the class of 2007 applied to advanced dental education programs, and of these 1,512 (90.5%) were accepted (159). Dental specialty training requires anything from one year to four-and-a-half years. Some specialties are very competitive; those applicants who are accepted typically have high dental school GPAs and NBDE scores.

Table A.7. Advanced Dental Education (35, 161)

Specialty	Average Post-Dental School Training in years	First-year residents enrolled in 2008	Total number of applications submitted[36]	Average first year resident net income (stipend – tuition & fees)	Median Gross Income of Practicing Specialist
Orthodonitcs & Dentofacial orthopedics	2.5	341	10,028	-11,347	$295,000
Pediatric Dentistry	2.1	349	7,716	18,620	$300,000
Periodontics	2.9	180	1,654	-1,557	$200,000
Prosthodontics	2.7	148	1,271	1,909	$190,820
Endodontics	2.2	202	3,776	-3,936	$394,120

[36] The number of individual applicants is not known and therefore the acceptance rate cannot be calculated. Most individual applicants submit multiple applications. The more competitive a specialty is, the more applications each applicant will submit.

Specialty	Average Post-Dental School Training in years	First-year residents enrolled in 2008	Total number of applications submitted[36]	Average first year resident net income (stipend – tuition & fees)	Median Gross Income of Practicing Specialist
Oral & Maxillofacial Pathology	3.1	12	67	21,176	
Oral & Maxillofacial Radiology	2.5	10	78	2,914	
Dental Public Health	1.2	22	57	10,810	
Oral and Maxillofacial Surgery	4.5	228	8,214	32,751	$400,000

Median gross income of general, non-specialist dentists who work full-time in a group practice: $220,000 (35)

Informative Websites

www.ada.org
www.adea.org
www.agd.org
www.braces.org
www.aaoms.org
www.aapd.org
www.perio.org
www.prosthodontics.org
www.aae.org
www.aaomr.org
www.aaphd.org

Audiologist (Au.D., CCC-A)

Doctor of Audiology, Certificate of Clinical Competence in Audiology

Description

Audiologists are autonomous practitioners who care for people with hearing, balance and other related ear problems. They examine patients, order diagnostic tests and interpret the results. They are trained to clean the ear canal, fit and dispense hearing aids, fit and tune cochlear implants and provide aural rehabilitation. Otolaryngologists (M.D.) place cochlear implants and perform surgery on the inner ear, and often work closely with audiologists.

Training

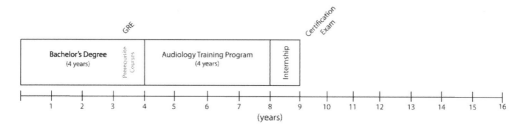

Audiologists first earn a bachelor's degree in any discipline and complete pre-requisite courses. Most programs require applicants to take the GRE in order to be considered for admission. Audiology training programs are four-year doctoral-degree programs that are accredited by the American Speech-Language-Hearing Association's (ASHA) Council on Academic Accreditation (CAA). After earning a doctorate in audiology, they must complete a 12-month internship. To become certified, audiologists must pass a certification exam. A Certificate of Clinical Competence in Audiology (CCC-A) is awarded by the ASHA and certification is awarded by the American Board of Audiology (ABA). In 2012, a doctoral degree will be required by the American Speech-Language-Hearing Association (ASHA) in order to earn the Certificate of Clinical Competence in Audiology (CCC-A).

Median Gross Income: $62,030 (137)

Informative Websites

www.asha.org
www.audiologist.org

Psychologist (Psy.D. or PhD)

Doctor of Psychology, Doctor of Philosophy in Psychology

Description

Psychologists assess, diagnose and treat individuals with mental disorders. Their treatment methods include individual psychotherapy, family therapy, group therapy and behavior modification programs. In most states, clinical psychologists are not allowed to prescribe medications. Psychiatrists, who are physicians (M.D. or D.O.) that have completed a residency in psychiatry, are the mental health professionals who can prescribe medications. Psychologists work at hospitals, clinics, universities, schools, government agencies and in industry.

Training

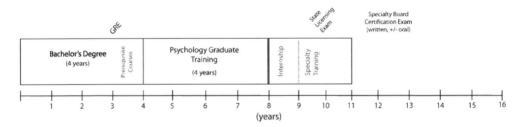

Psychologists first earn a bachelor's degree in any discipline. They then go on to earn a doctoral degree, Psy.D. or PhD in psychology. After earning their doctorate, they must complete an internship before they may practice independently. The American Psychological Association (APA) accredits doctoral training programs and internship programs. Certification and licensing requirements vary among states. Most states require one to two years of professional experience as well as successfully passing a certification examination.

The American Board of Professional Psychology (ABPP) recognizes professional achievement by awarding specialty certification in the following specialties.

- Cinical Child & Adolescent Psychology
- Clinical Health Psychology
- Clinical Neuropsychology
- Clinical Psychology
- Cognitive & Behavioral Psychology
- Counseling Psychology
- Couple & Family Psychology
- Forensic Psychology

- Group Psychology
- Organizational & Business Consulting Psychology
- Psychoanalysis in Psychology
- Rehabilitation Psychology
- School Psychology

To earn ABPP specialty certification, psychologists must have a doctorate in psychology, hold an active state license, complete the training requirements for that specialty and successfully pass specialty board exams.

Median Gross Income: $64,140 (117)

Informative Websites

www.apa.org
www.aacpsy.org
www.abpp.org

Podiatrist (D.P.M.)

Doctor of Podiatric Medicine

Description

Podiatrists diagnose and treat diseases, disorders and injuries of the foot and ankle. They may prescribe medications, orthotics or physical therapy. Podiatrists may also perform surgery on the foot and lower leg.

Training

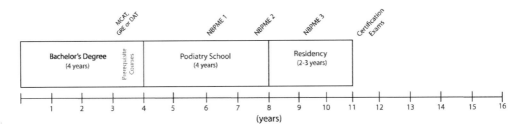

To become a podiatrist one must complete at least 3 years of undergraduate course-work; however, about 95% of podiatry students earn a bachelor's degree prior to starting podiatry school(118). To be considered for admission, applicants must take the MCAT, DAT or GRE. Podiatry school is four years long. In order to become licensed, most states require at least two years of residency training and passing scores on the National Board of Podiatric Medical Examiners (NBPME) parts one, two and three exams. Podiatric residency programs last from two to three years. Two-year programs lead to certification in foot surgery by the American Board of Podiatric Surgery (ABPS) and American Board of Podiatric Orthopedics and Primary Podiatric Medicine (ABPOPPM). Three-year programs offer more training in reconstructive rear foot and ankle surgery and lead to certification in foot surgery and reconstructive rear foot and ankle surgery by the American Board of Podiatric Surgery (ABPS) and the American Board of Podiatric Orthopedics and Primary Podiatric Medicine (ABPOPPM). Podiatry schools and residencies are accredited by the Council on Podiatric Medical Education (CPME) of the American Podiatric Medical Association (APMA).

Table A.8.   *Podiatric Medicine - 2009 Incoming Class(162-164)*

Applicants	976
Matriculants	579
Matriculation Rate	59%
Matriculant Average Undergraduate GPA	3.3
Matriculant Average MCAT score	22.1

Median Gross Income: $113,650 (118)

Informative Websites

www.apma.org
www.aacpm.org

Oral Surgeon (D.D.S. +/- M.D.)

Doctor of Dental Surgery, Medicinae Doctor[37]
Also known as: Oral & Maxillofacial Surgeon

Description

Oral surgeons diagnose and surgically treat diseases, defects and injuries involving the hard and soft tissues of the oral and maxillofacial region. They extract problematic wisdom teeth, align misaligned jaws, treat facial fractures, remove tumors and place dental implants.

Training

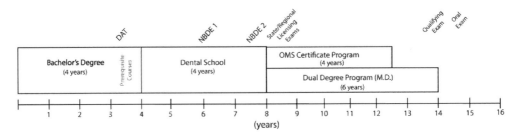

To become an oral surgeon, one must graduate from dental school and complete an oral and maxillofacial surgery training program. This training includes extensive experience in oral and maxillofacial surgery as well as clinical rotations in general surgery, internal medicine, anesthesia and pathology.

An oral & maxillofacial surgery (OMFS) certificate can be earned after completing a four-year training program. Dual-degree programs are around six-years in length and integrate medical school curriculum with the OMFS training. Graduates of six-year programs are awarded an M.D. in addition to their OMFS certificate. Dentists in dual-degree programs also take the USMLE steps 1, 2 and 3. To become board certified, oral surgeons must pass a written qualifying exam and an oral certification exam following their residency training.

In 2007, 58% of applicants were accepted into oral and maxillofacial surgery training programs (165). Programs are accredited by the Commission on Dental Accreditation (CODA).

Median Gross Income: $400,000 (35)

---

[37] M.D. is an acronym which stands for the Latin "Medicinae Doctor." In the United States M.D. is interpreted as Medical Doctor and refers to the allopathic type of physician.

Informative Websites

www.aboms.org
www.omsfoundation.org
www.natmatch.com
www.aaoms.org

Physician (M.D. or D.O.)

Medicinae Doctor, Doctor of Osteopathic Medicine
Also known as: Doctor, Doctor of Medicine, Doctor of Osteopathic Medicine

Description

Physicians diagnose and treat disease and injury of the entire body. Physicians also provide supportive care to patients with incurable diseases in an effort to maximize their quality of life and minimize suffering. The diagnostic process typically begins with the physician obtaining a history by way of a conversation with a patient. The history is followed by a physical examination of the patient's body. After the history and physical exam, a physician may order and/or perform tests to help them make a diagnosis. After making a diagnosis they will counsel patients and discuss available medications and/or procedures to help treat their disease or injury. With the patient's consent, physicians may then prescribe medications, perform surgery or consult other physicians.

Education and Training

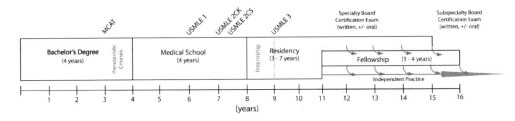

The road to becoming a licensed and board certified physician is a long, complicated and expensive one. It can take anywhere from 11 to 16 years of overtime[38] training after high school – or more, if one takes time off along the way.

To become a physician one must earn a bachelor's degree, which typically takes 4 years. Acceptance to medical school is notoriously competitive, so college students interested in going to medical school usually study more than their peers who are not interested in going to medical school. In 2008, 42,269 people applied to U.S. allopathic medical schools for the entering class of 2009; however, there were only 18,390 training positions (8). Therefore, 56.5% of those who applied were not given the opportunity to attend a U.S. allopathic medical school. The medical school application process is explained in chapter 11. Statistics of those who were accepted to medical school are explained in chapter 9.

---

[38] Full-time refers to 40 hours per week. Most medical students, residents and fellows spend nearly 80 hours per week caring for patients and studying.

For most people, medical school is not easy. Most medical students report spending 70+ hours per week on medical school activities such as studying, attending lectures and working in the hospital. Those who are accepted into U.S. allopathic medical schools will probably graduate, as 96% of matriculants graduate within 10 years, with most graduating in four years (8).

Medical school is expensive. For the 2009-2010 academic year, the median cost of tuition and fees for public and private medical schools was $24,384 and $43,002 per year respectively (16). This does not include the cost of rent, utilities, food, transportation, health insurance, books, professional attire, licensing exams or residency interview expenses. Most medical students borrow an additional $15,000 - $20,000 per year to cover these expenses. For more information on life in medical school, see chapter 12. For more information on the finances of becoming a physician, see chapter 5.

After medical school, graduates move on to residency. Depending on the specialty, residency can take from 3 to 7 years to complete. The first year of residency is known as internship. To become board certified, one must complete a residency and pass all additional exams for that particular specialty. For example, to become a board certified Internal Medicine physician - one must graduate from medical school, pass all USMLEs, complete a 3-year internal medicine residency and pass the internal medicine board exam. To become a board certified Thoracic Surgeon, one must graduate from medical school, pass all USMLEs, complete a 5-year general surgery residency, complete a 2-year thoracic surgery fellowship and pass the thoracic surgery board exams. Like medical school, residency is not easy. Most residents approach the legal work-hour limit of 80 hours per week throughout their residency. Residents do not have to pay tuition, and make about $50,000 per year, or $12.50 per hour.

In the United States, physicians can practice medicine independently after passing all USMLEs and completing an internship; however, they will not be board certified in any specialty. It is extremely rare for a physician to start practicing medicine independently after their internship, without completing a residency program and becoming board certified. Most people prefer to be cared for by a physician who is board certified. Physicians who are not board certified may find it difficult to obtain malpractice insurance or hospital privileges.

In the United States, there are over 25,000 residency-training positions available each year. Note that there are almost 10,000 more residency-training positions available each year than the number of U.S. allopathic medical students who graduate each year. In 2009 the National Residency Matching Program (NRMP) enrolled 4,299 programs which offered 25,185 training positions (72). 95.4% of these positions were filled (73). A total of 35,972 applicants participated in the match (72). 15,638 were U.S. allopathic medical school seniors (28). 1,222 were former graduates of U.S. Medical Schools (28). 2,013 were students or graduates of osteopathic medical schools (28). 3,390 were U.S. citizens who graduated from International Medical Schools (28). 7,484 were non-U.S.

citizen graduates of International Medical Schools (28). The overall residency match rate among all applicants in 2009 was 71.4% (73). U.S. allopathic medical school seniors were most successful in landing a residency position with a 93.1% match rate (73). For more information regarding the varying competitiveness among different specialties and the residency matching process, see chapter 16.

Median gross income varies greatly by specialty. For median incomes by specialty see Table 13.1.

Informative Websites

www.aamc.org/students
www.ama-assn.org/go/becominganmd
www.fsmb.org
www.osteopathic.org
www.ambs.org
www.facs.org

Appendix 2   Acronyms

AA-C	Anesthesia Assistant Certified
AADSAS	Associated American Dental Schools Application Service
AAMC	Association of American Medical Colleges
AAMFT	American Association for Marriage and Family Therapy
ABA	American Board of Audiology
ABC	American Board for Certification
ABGC	American Board of Genetic Counseling
ABHES	Accrediting Bureau of Health Education Schools
ABMS	American Board of Medical Specialties
ABO	American Board of Opticianry
ABPOPPM	American Board of Podiatric Orthopedics and Primary Podiatric Medicine
ABPP	American Board of Professional Psychology
ABPS	American Board of Podiatric Surgery
ABRET	American Board of Registration of Electroencephalographic and Evoked Potential Technologists
ABS	Applied Basic Science exam
ACLS	Advanced Cardiac Life Support
ACME	Accreditation Commission for Midwifery Education
ACNM	American College of Nurse-Midwives
ACNP	Acute Care Nurse Practitioner
ACOTE	Accreditation Council for Occupational Therapy Education
ACPE	Accreditation Council for Pharmacy Education
ADA	American Dietetic Association
ADN	Associates Degree in Nursing
AED	Automated External Defibrillator
AIDS	Acquired Immunodeficiency Syndrome
AKA	American Kinesiotherapy Association
AMA	American Medical Association
AMT	American Medical Technologists
ANCC	American Nurses Credentialing Center
ANP	Adult Nurse Practitioner
APA	American Psychological Association
APMA	American Podiatric Medical Association
ARC-PA	Accreditation Review Commission on Education for the Physician Assistant
ARDMS	American Registry of Diagnostic Medical Sonographers
ARRT	American Registry of Radiologic Technologists
ASCP	American Society for Clinical Pathology
ASHA	American Speech-Language-Hearing Association
ASPT	American Society for Phlebotomy Technicians
ASSH	American Society for Surgery of the Hand
AUA	American Urological Association
AuD	Doctor of Audiology

BA	Bachelor of Arts
BOC	Board Of Certification
BS	Bachelor of Science
BSN	Bachelor of Science in Nursing
BSW	Bachelors degree in Social Work
CAA	Council on Academic Accreditation
CAAHEP	Commission on Accreditation of Allied Health Education Programs
CABG	Coronary Artery Bypass Grafting
CADE	Commission on Accreditation for Dietetics Education
CAP	Clinical Applications in Perfusion
CAPTE	Commission on Accreditation of Physical Therapy Education
CASPA	Central Application Service for Physician Assistants
CCC-A	Certificate of Clinical Competence in Audiology
CCC-SLP	Certificate of Clinical Competency in Speech and Language Pathology
CCE	Council on Chiropractic Education
CCI	Cardiovascular Credentialing International
CCNA	Council on Certification of Nurse Anesthetists
CCNE	Commission on Collegiate Nursing Education
CCP	Certified Clinical Perfusionist
CDA	Certified Dental Assistant
CDT	Certified Dental laboratory Technician
CFA	Certified First Assistant
CLC	Child Life Council
CM	Certified Midwife
CM	Case Manager
CMA	Certified Medical Assistant
CNA	Certified Nurse Assistant
CNM	Certified Nurse Midwife
CNMT	Certified Nuclear Medicine Technologist
CNS	Clinical Nurse Specialist
COAMFTE	Commission on Accreditation for Marriage and Family Therapy Education
CoARC	Committee on Accreditation for Respiratory Care
CODA	Commission on Dental Accreditation
COPD	Chronic Obstructive Pulmonary Disease
CPhT	Certified Pharmacy Technician
CPME	Council on Podiatric Medical Education
CPO	Certified Prosthetist and Orthotist
CPR	Cardiopulmonary Resuscitation
CPT	Certified Phlebotomy Technician
CRNA	Certified Registered Nurse Anesthetist
CSA	Certified Surgical Assistant
CSE	Clinical Skills Exam
CST	Certified Surgical Technologist
CSWE	Council on Social Work Education
CT	Computed Tomography
DANB	Dental Assisting National Board
DAT	Dental Admissions Test

DC	Doctor of Chiropractic
DDS	Doctor of Dental Surgery
DM	Diabetes Mellitus
DMD	Doctor Dental Medicine
DNA	Deoxyribonucleic Acid
DO	Doctor of Osteopathic Medicine
DPM	Doctor of Podiatric Medicine
DPT	Doctor of Physical Therapy
EEG	Electroencephalogram
EMT	Emergency Medical Technician
EP	Evoked Potential studies
ERAS	Electronic Residency Application Service
FMG	Foreign Medical Graduate
FNP	Family Nurse Practitioner
FRIEDA	Fellowship and Residency Electronic Interactive Database Access System
GED	General Equivalency Diploma
GNP	Geriatric Nurse Practitioner
GPA	Grade Point Average
GRE	Graduate Record Examination
HD	Hemodialysis
HIV	Human Immunodeficiency Virus
HPERB	Health Professions Education Requirement Board
HPSP	Health Professions Scholarship Program
HT	Histotechnician
IMG	International Medical Graduate
IONP	Intra-operative neuromonitoring
IV	Intravenous
JSGMEB	Joint Service Graduate Medical Education Selection Board
LCWS	Licensed Clinical Social Worker
LPC	Licensed Professional Counselor
LPN	Licensed Practical Nurse
LPT	Licensed Physical Therapist
LRT	Licensed Respiratory Therapist
LTM	Long Term Monitoring (electroencephalogram)
LVN	Licensed Vocational Nurse
MCAT	Medical College Admissions Test
MD	Medicinae Doctor (Latin for 'Doctor of Medicine')
MLT	Medical Laboratory Technician
MPH	Master of Public Health
MPJE	Multistate Pharmacy Jurisprudence Exam
MRI	Magnetic Resonance Imaging
MS	Master of Science
MSN	Master of Science in Nursing
MSW	Masters degree in Social Work
NAACLS	National Accrediting Agency for Clinical Laboratory Sciences
NAPLEX	North American Pharmacist Licensure Exam
NATA	National Athletic Trainers' Association

NBCE	National Board of Chiropractic Examiners
NBDE	National Board of Dental Examiners
NBEO	National Board of Examiners in Optometry
NBME	National Board of Medical Examiners
NBPME	National Board of Podiatric Medical Examiners
NBRC	National Board for Respiratory Care
NBSTSA	National Board of Surgical Technology and Surgical Assisting
NCCAA	National Commission for Certification of Anesthesiologist Assistants
NCCPA	National Commission on Certification of Physician Assistants
NCE	National Certification Exam
NCLE	National Contact Lens Examiners
NCLEX-PN	National Council Licensure Examination for Practical Nurses
NCLEX-RN	National Council Licensure Examination for Registered Nurses
NCMHCE	National Certified Mental Health Counselor Examination
NCOPE	National Commission on Orthotic and Prosthetic Education
NCS	Nerve Conduction Studies
NHTSA	National Highway Traffic Safety Administration
NLNAC	National League for Nursing Accrediting Commission
NMTCB	Nuclear Medicine Technology Certification Board
NNP	Neonatal Nurse Practitioner
NP	Nurse Practitioner
NP-C	Nurse Practitioner - Certified
NPTE	National Physical Therapy Examination
NREMT	National Registry of Emergency Medical Technicians
NRMP	National Residency Matching Program
OAT	Optometry Admissions Test
OD	Oculis Doctor (Latin for 'Doctor of Optometry')
OMFS	Oral and Maxillofacial Surgery
ONP	Oncology Nurse Practitioner
OTR	Occupational Therapist Registered
PA	Physician's Assistant
PA-C	Physician's Assistant - Certified
PAM	Patient Assessment and Management exam
PANCE	Physician Assistant National Certifying Examination
PCAT	Pharmacy College Admission Test
PGY-1	Post Graduate Year one (a first-year resident = intern)
PGY-5	A resident or fellow in their fifth year of post medical school training
PharmD	Doctor of Pharmacy
PhD	Doctor of Philosophy
PMHNP	Psychiatry and Mental Health Nurse Practitioner
PNP	Pediatric Nurse Practitioner
PSG	Polysomnogram
PsyD	Doctor of Psychology
PT	Physical Therapist
PTCE	Pharmacy Technician Certification Exam
R.Ph.	Registered Pharmacist
RD	Registered Dietician

RDH	Registered Dental Hygienist
RDMS	Registered Diagnostic Medical Sonographer
RN	Registered Nurse
RNA	Ribonucleic Acid
RPT	Registered Phlebotomy Technician
RPT	Registered Physical Therapist
RRT	Registered Respiratory Therapist
USMLE	United States Medical Licensing Examination
WHNP	Women's Health Nurse Practitioner

References

1.   OECD Health Data 2009: Statistics and Indicators for 30 Countries. Washington DC, 2009.

2.   U.S. Department of Labor, Career Guide to Industries. *Healthcare*, 2010-11 Edition Ed: Bureau of Labor Statistics.

3.   Period Life Table. Social Security Online, 2006.

4.   Matriculating Student Questionaire (MSQ) 2009 All Schools Report. 2009.

5.   GQ Medical School Graduation Questionnaire FINAL All Schools Summary Report 2009.

6.   Total Student Budgets, 2009-2010. *Trends in Higher Education*: The College Board, Annual Survey of Colleges, 2009. P. Figure 1.

7.   Schools Offering Combined Degree Programs in BS/MD Vol. 2010: Association of American Medical Colleges 2010.

8.   U.S. Medical School Applicants and Students 1982-83 to 2009-10. AAMC, 2009.

9.   Table 18: MCAT and GPAs for Applicants and Matriculants to U.S. Medical Schools by Primary Undergraduate Major, 2009. Association of American Medical Colleges, 2009.

10.   AACOMAS Matriculant Profile of 2009 Entering Class. Chevy Chase, MD, 2009.

11.   AACOMAS Applicant Pool Profile 2009 Entering Class. Chevy Chase, MD, 2009.

12.   Kleshinski, J., Khuder, S. A., Shapiro, J. I., et al. Impact of preadmission variables on USMLE step 1 and step 2 performance. *Adv Health Sci Educ Theory Pract* 14: 69-78, 2009.

13.   Time Paradigm. Dictionary.com, 2009.

14.   DeNavas-Walt, C., Proctor, B. D., Smith, J. C. Income, Poverty, and Health Insurance Coverage in the United States: 2007. *Current Population Reports*. Washington, DC: U.S. Census Bureau, 2008. P. 6.

15.   2008-09 Survey of Dental Education. *Tuition, Admission, and Attrition*, Vol. 2. Chicago, 2009.

16.   U.S. Medical Schools Tuition and Student Fees - First Year Students 2009-2010 And 2008-2009. 2010.

17.   Anim, M., Markert, R. J., Wood, V. C., et al. Physician practice patterns resemble ACGME duty hours. *Am J Med* 122: 587-593, 2009.

18.   Gibbs, R. S. *Danforth's Obstetrics and Gynecology*, 10 Ed. Philadelphia PA: Lippincott Williams & Wilkins, 2008.

19.   Dunson, D. B., Baird, D. D., Colombo, B. Increased infertility with age in men and women. *Obstet Gynecol* 103: 51-56, 2004.

20.   Heffner, L. J. Advanced maternal age--how old is too old? *N Engl J Med* 351: 1927-1929, 2004.

21.   Menken, J., Trussell, J., Larsen, U. Age and infertility. *Science* 233: 1389-1394, 1986.

22.   Gindoff, P. R., Jewelewicz, R. Reproductive potential in the older woman. *Fertil Steril* 46: 989-1001, 1986.

23. Morris, J. K., Mutton, D. E., Alberman, E. Revised estimates of the maternal age specific live birth prevalence of Down's syndrome. *J Med Screen* 9: 2-6, 2002.

24. Hook, E. B., Cross, P. K., Schreinemachers, D. M. Chromosomal abnormality rates at amniocentesis and in live-born infants. *JAMA* 249: 2034-2038, 1983.

25. Creasy, Resnick. *Maternal Fetal Medicine: Practice and Principles*. Philadelphia: W.B. Saunders, 1994.

26. Ron-El, R., Raziel, A., Strassburger, D., et al. Outcome of assisted reproductive technology in women over the age of 41. *Fertil Steril* 74: 471-475, 2000.

27. Stromberg, B., Dahlquist, G., Ericson, A., et al. Neurological sequelae in children born after in-vitro fertilisation: a population-based study. *Lancet* 359: 461-465, 2002.

28. NRMP. Charting Outcomes in the Match. 3rd Ed. Washington, DC, 2009.

29. AAMC Survey of Resident/Fellow Stipends and Benefits. *Health Care Affairs*, 2009.

30. 2009 Physician Compensation Survey. Alexandria, VA, 2009.

31. Service, I. R. IRS Publication 15 (Circular E), Employer's Tax Guide. In D. o. t. Treasury (Ed.). Washington, DC, 2010. P. 40.

32. Publication 15 Cat. No. 10000W. In Treasury (Ed.): Internal Revenue Service, 2010. P. 40.

33. Dorsey, E. R., Jarjoura, D., Rutecki, G. W. Influence of controllable lifestyle on recent trends in specialty choice by US medical students. *JAMA* 290: 1173-1178, 2003.

34. Shiotani, L. M., Parkerton, P. H., Wenger, N. S., et al. Internal medicine work hours: trends, associations, and implications for the future. *Am J Med* 121: 80-85, 2008.

35. Income from the Private Practice of Dentistry. *2008 Survey of Dental Practice*, Vol. 3: American Dental Association, 2009.

36. Occupational Outlook Handbook, 2010-2011 Edition, Teachers—Kindergarten, Elementary, Middle, and Secondary. Bureau of Labor and Statistics, U.S. Department of Labor, 2010.

37. Occupational Outlook Handbook, 2010-2011 Edition, Registered Nurses. Bureau of Labor and Statistics, U.S. Department of Labor, 2010.

38. National Health Service Corps. U.S. Department of Health and Human Services, 2010.

39. Indian Health Service. U.S. Department of Health and Human Services, 2010.

40. Freedom to persue your career in research. U.S. Department of Health and Human services, 2010.

41. Fiscal Year 2009 Highlights. U.S. Department of Health and Human Sevices - National Institutes of Health, 2009.

42. Cole, P. A. NIH Intramural Loan Repayment Program Fiscal Year 2008 Highlights. U.S. Department of Health and Human Services - National Institutes of Health, 2008.

43. Basic Eligibility Requirements. Vol. 2010: U.S. Department of Health and Human Services, 2010.

44. Recruitment. Uniformed Services University of the Health Sciences, 2009.

45. Christensen, K. L. Military Graduate Medical Education. 2010.

46. Landon, B. E., Reschovsky, J. D., Pham, H. H., et al. Leaving medicine: the consequences of physician dissatisfaction. *Med Care* 44: 234-242, 2006.

47. Landon, B. E., Reschovsky, J., Blumenthal, D. Changes in career satisfaction among primary care and specialist physicians, 1997-2001. *JAMA* 289: 442-449, 2003.
48. Boukus, E., Cassil, A., O'Malley, A. S. A Snapshot of U.S. Physicians: Key Findings from the 2008 Health Tracking Physician Survey. Vol. 35. Washington, DC, 2009.
49. U.S. Job Satisfaction at Lowest Level in Two Decades. The Conference Board, 2010.
50. U.S Job Satisfaction Declines, The Conference Board Reports. The Conference Board, 2007.
51. Leigh, J. P., Tancredi, D. J., Kravitz, R. L. Physician career satisfaction within specialties. *BMC Health Serv Res* 9: 166, 2009.
52. Frank, E., McMurray, J. E., Linzer, M., et al. Career satisfaction of US women physicians: results from the Women Physicians' Health Study. Society of General Internal Medicine Career Satisfaction Study Group. *Arch Intern Med* 159: 1417-1426, 1999.
53. Clark, A., Oswald, A. Satisfaction and comparision income. *Journal of Public Economics* 61: 359-381, 1996.
54. Haas, J. S., Cook, E. F., Puopolo, A. L., et al. Is the professional satisfaction of general internists associated with patient satisfaction? *J Gen Intern Med* 15: 122-128, 2000.
55. *Physician Specialty Data: A Chart Book*: Association of American Medical Colleges, 2006.
56. OMT: Hands-On Care. American Osteopathic Association, 2010.
57. Association, A. O. Osteopathic Medicine. Vol. 2010, 2010.
58. Liaison Committee on Medical Education. 2010.
59. 2010 AOA Intern/Resident Registration Program Amerian Osteopathic Association, 2010.
60. Physician Education, Licensure, and Certification. Vol. 2010: American Medical Association, 2005.
61. Table 17: MCAT Scores and GPAs for Applicants and Matriculants to U.S. Medical Schools, 1998-2009. Association of American Medical Colleges, 2009.
62. 2008 USMLE Performance Data. *2008 NBME Annual Report*, 2009.
63. ACT Profile Report - National. 2009.
64. Ziomek, R. L. Request for data about ACT test takers In B. J. Brown (Ed.): Department of Education and Workforce Research Services, 2010.
65. 2009 College-Bound Seniors Total Group Profile Report. The College Board, 2009.
66. ACT and SAT Concordance Tables. New York, 2009.
67. Membership. Association of American Medical Colleges, 2010.
68. Age of Applicants to U.S. Medical Schools at Anticipated Matriculation by Sex and Race and Ethnicity, 2006-2009. 2009.
69. Member Colleges. American Association of College of Osteopathic Medicine, 2010.
70. Table 6: Age of Applicants to U.S. Medical Schools at Anticipated Matriculation by Sex and Race and Ethnicity. Association of American Medical Colleges, 2009.
71. Levitan, T. A Report on a Survey of Osteopathic Medical School Growth, 2007-08. Chevy Chase, 2008.
72. About NRMP. National Resident Matching Program, 2010.

73. Program, N. R. M. Results and Data: 2009 Main Residency Match. Washington, DC, 2009.

74. 2010 MCAT Essentials. *Association of American Medical Colleges.* Washington, DC, 2010.

75. Julian, E. R. Validity of the Medical College Admission Test for predicting medical school performance. *Acad Med* 80: 910-917, 2005.

76. Donnon, T., Paolucci, E. O., Violato, C. The predictive validity of the MCAT for medical school performance and medical board licensing examinations: a meta-analysis of the published research. *Acad Med* 82: 100-106, 2007.

77. Basco, W. T., Jr., Way, D. P., Gilbert, G. E., et al. Undergraduate institutional MCAT scores as predictors of USMLE step 1 performance. *Acad Med* 77: S13-16, 2002.

78. Veloski, J. J., Callahan, C. A., Xu, G., et al. Prediction of students' performances on licensing examinations using age, race, sex, undergraduate GPAs, and MCAT scores. *Acad Med* 75: S28-30, 2000.

79. Evans, P., Wen, F. K. Does the medical college admission test predict global academic performance in osteopathic medical school? *J Am Osteopath Assoc* 107: 157-162, 2007.

80. Hughes, P. Can we improve on how we select medical students? *J R Soc Med* 95: 18-22, 2002.

81. Table 32: MD-PhD Applicants, Acceptees, Matriculants, and Graduates of U.S. Medical Schools by sex 1999-2009. Association of American Medical Colleges, 2009.

82. Table 35: MCAT Scores and GPAs for MD/PhD Applicants and Matriculants to U.S. Medical Schools, 2008-2009.: Association of American Medical Colleges, 2009.

83. Janis, J. E., Hatef, D. A. Resident selection protocols in plastic surgery: a national survey of plastic surgery program directors. *Plast Reconstr Surg* 122: 1929-1939; discussion 1940-1921, 2008.

84. AMCAS 2010 Instructions. Association of American Medical Colleges, 2009.

85. Examination Fees. National Board of Medical Examiners, 2010.

86. Minimum Passing Scores on USMLE Step Examinations. USMLE, 2010.

87. USMLE 2010 Bulletin of Information. Federation of State Medical Boards of the United States, Inc., and the National Board of Medical Examiners, 2009.

88. How Members are Chosen. Alpha Omega Alpha Honor Medical Society, 2009.

89. What Board Certification Means. American Board of Medical Specialties, 2010.

90. Dorsey, E. R., Jarjoura, D., Rutecki, G. W. The influence of controllable lifestyle and sex on the specialty choices of graduating U.S. medical students, 1996-2003. *Acad Med* 80: 791-796, 2005.

91. Rates, Withholding Schedules, and Meals and Lodging Values. State of California, 2010.

92. Training Options. American Board of Medical Genetics, 2010.

93. Certification and Requirements. American Board of Nuclear Medicine, 2010.

94. Certification Requirements. American Board of Preventative Medicine, 2010.

95. Subspecialties. American Board of Preventative Medicine, 2010.

96. Burkhart, D. N., Lischka, T. A. Dual and parallel postdoctoral training programs: implications for the osteopathic medical profession. *J Am Osteopath Assoc* 109: 146-153, 2009.

97. Crosby, J. Osteopathic Match Results Released. *Daily Report Blog*: American Osteopathic Association, 2009.

98. Freeman, E., Lischka, T. A. Osteopathic graduate medical education. *J Am Osteopath Assoc* 109: 135-145,196-138, 2009.

99. Burkhart, D. N., Lischka, T. A. Osteopathic graduate medical education. *J Am Osteopath Assoc* 108: 127-137, 2008.

100. Urology Match Statistics. American Urological Association, 2009.

101. Ophthalmology Residency Match Report – January 2009. San Francisco, 2009.

102. Child Neurology & Neurodevelopmental Disability Residency Match Comparative Statistics. San Francisco, 2009.

103. 2010 Match Results. DO-online.org, 2010.

104. NRMP. Results and Data: Specialties Matching Service 2009 Appointment Year. Washington, DC, 2009.

105. Fellowship Match. San Fransisco: San Fransisco Matching Programs, 2010.

106. Certified Nursing Assistant - Median Base salary. Salary.com, 2010.

107. Occupational Outlook Handbook, 2010-2011 Edition, Clinical Labratory Technologists and Technicians. Bureau of Labor and Statistics, U.S. Department of Labor, 2010.

108. Emergency Medical Technician (Basic) - Base salary. Salary.com, 2010.

109. Emergency Medical Technician - Paramedic. Clearwater, FL: Commission on Accreditation of Allied Health Programs, 2009.

110. Occupational Outlook Handbook, 2010-2011 Edition, Pharmacy Technicians and Aides. Bureau of Labor and Statistics, U.S. Department of Labor, 2010.

111. Occupational Outlook Handbook, 2010-2011 Edition, Surgical Technologists. Bureau of Labor and Statistics, U.S. Department of Labor, 2010.

112. Occupational Outlook Handbook, 2010-2011 Edition, Speech-Language Pathologists. Bureau of Labor and Statistics, U.S. Department of Labor, 2010.

113. Occupational Outlook Handbook, 2010-2011 Edition, Social Workers. Bureau of Labor and Statistics, U.S. Department of Labor, 2010.

114. Occupational Outlook Handbook, 2010-2011 Edition, Respiratory Therapists. Bureau of Labor and Statistics, U.S. Department of Labor, 2010.

115. Occupational Outlook Handbook, 2010-2011 Edition, Radiologic Technologists and Technicians. Bureau of Labor and Statistics, U.S. Department of Labor, 2010.

116. Occupational Outlook Handbook, 2010-2011 Edition, Radiation Therapists. Bureau of Labor and Statistics, U.S. Department of Labor, 2010.

117. Occupational Outlook Handbook, 2010-2011 Edition, Psychologists. Bureau of Labor and Statistics, U.S. Department of Labor, 2010.

118. Occupational Outlook Handbook, 2010-2011 Edition, Podiatrists. Bureau of Labor and Statistics, U.S. Department of Labor, 2010.

119. Occupational Outlook Handbook, 2010-2011 Edition, Physician Assistants. Bureau of Labor and Statistics, U.S. Department of Labor, 2010.
120. Occupational Outlook Handbook, 2010-2011 Edition, Physical Therapists. Bureau of Labor and Statistics, U.S. Department of Labor, 2010.
121. Occupational Outlook Handbook, 2010-2011 Edition, Pharmacists. Bureau of Labor and Statistics, U.S. Department of Labor, 2010.
122. Occupational Outlook Handbook, 2010-2011 Edition, Optometrists. Bureau of Labor and Statistics, U.S. Department of Labor, 2010.
123. Occupational Outlook Handbook, 2010-2011 Edition, Opticians, Dispensing. Bureau of Labor and Statistics, U.S. Department of Labor, 2010.
124. Occupational Outlook Handbook, 2010-2011 Edition, Occupational Therapists. Bureau of Labor and Statistics, U.S. Department of Labor, 2010.
125. Occupational Outlook Handbook, 2010-2011 Edition, Nuclear Medicine Technologists. Bureau of Labor and Statistics, U.S. Department of Labor, 2010.
126. Occupational Outlook Handbook, 2010-2011 Edition, Medical, Dental, and Ophthalmic Labratory Technicians. Bureau of Labor and Statistics, U.S. Department of Labor, 2010.
127. Occupational Outlook Handbook, 2010-2011 Edition, Medical Assistants. Bureau of Labor and Statistics, U.S. Department of Labor, 2010.
128. Occupational Outlook Handbook, 2010-2011 Edition, Licensed Practical and Licensed Vocational Nurses. Bureau of Labor and Statistics, U.S. Department of Labor, 2010.
129. Occupational Outlook Handbook, 2010-2011 Edition, Dietitians and Nutritionists. Bureau of Labor and Statistics, U.S. Department of Labor, 2010.
130. Occupational Outlook Handbook, 2010-2011 Edition, Diagnostic Medical Sonographers. Bureau of Labor and Statistics, U.S. Department of Labor, 2010.
131. Occupational Outlook Handbook, 2010-2011 Edition, Dentists. Bureau of Labor and Statistics, U.S. Department of Labor, 2010.
132. Occupational Outlook Handbook, 2010-2011 Edition, Dental Hygienists. Bureau of Labor and Statistics, U.S. Department of Labor, 2010.
133. Occupational Outlook Handbook, 2010-2011 Edition, Dental Assistants. Bureau of Labor and Statistics, U.S. Department of Labor, 2010.
134. Occupational Outlook Handbook, 2010-2011 Edition, Counselors. Bureau of Labor and Statistics, U.S. Department of Labor, 2010.
135. Occupational Outlook Handbook, 2010-2011 Edition, Chiropractors. Bureau of Labor and Statistics, U.S. Department of Labor, 2010.
136. Occupational Outlook Handbook, 2010-2011 Edition, Cardiovascular Technologists and Technicians.: Bureau of Labor and Statistics, U.S. Department of Labor, 2010.
137. Occupational Outlook Handbook, 2010-2011 Edition, Audiologists. Bureau of Labor and Statistics, U.S. Department of Labor, 2010.
138. Occupational Outlook Handbook, 2010-2011 Edition, Athletic Trainers. Bureau of Labor and Statistics, U.S. Department of Labor, 2010.
139. Electroneurodiagnostic Technologist - Base salary. Salary.com, 2010.

140. Summary of the 2008 Child Life Profession Compensation Survey Results. Rockville, MD, 2009.

141. Cardio-Pulmonary Perfusionist - Base salary. Salary.com, 2010.

142. Average Technologist Molecular Genetics Salaries in New York, NY. simplyhired.com, 2010.

143. Cytogenetic Technologist - Base salary. Salary.com, 2010.

144. Genetic Counselor - Median Base salary. Salary.com, 2010.

145. Salary Survey for Degree: MPH. *Median Salary by Job, Degree: MPH*: Payscale.com, 2010.

146. Prosthetist/Orthotist - Median Base salary. Salary.com, 2010.

147. Clinical Nurse Specialist - Base salary. Salary.com, 2010.

148. Certified Nurse Midwife - Median Base salary. Salary.com, 2010.

149. Licensed Professional Counselor - Median Base salary. Salary.com, 2010.

150. Nurse Practitioner - Median Base salary. Salary.com, 2010.

151. Nurse Anesthetist - Median Base salary. Salary.com, 2010.

152. Paramedic - Median Base salary. Salary.com, 2010.

153. 2008-09 Survey of Allied Dental Education. Chicago, 2009.

154. Association, A. M. *Health Care Careers Directory, 2009-2010*. Chicago: American Medical Association Press, 2009.

155. McDaniel, M. J. The Applicant Pool 2008-2009 Cycle 8 Report. In *Annual Education Forum*, Portland, 2009.

156. Prospective Students. The Association of Chiropractic Colleges, 2010.

157. Calculated from Profile of 2009 Entering Class. Rockville: Association of Schools and Colleges of Optometry, 2009.

158. Zuckerman, J. Request for Data. In B. Brown (Ed.), 2010.

159. 2008-09 Survey of Dental Education. *Academic Programs, Enrollment, and Graduates*, Vol. 1. Chicago, 2010.

160. *Dental Admission Test (DAT) 2010 Program Guide*. Chicago: American Dental Association, 2009.

161. 2008-09 Survey of Advanced Dental Education. Chicago, 2010.

162. Matriculant GPA Averages by Year. Rockville MD: American Association of Colleges of Podiatric Medicine, 2009.

163. Matriculant MCAT Averages by Year. Rockville MD: American Association of Colleges of Podiatric Medicine, 2009.

164. Applicant GPA Averages by Year. Rockville MD: American Association of Colleges of Podiatric Medicine, 2009.

165. Explore a Future in Oral and Maxillofacial Surgery. Rosemont, IL: American Association of Oral and Maxillofacial Surgeons, 2010.

Made in the USA
San Bernardino, CA
08 September 2016